AGEING, NUTRITION AND HEALTH

AGEING, NUTRITION AND HEALTH

Pallavi M. Mehta
Komal B. Chauhan

KALPAZ

ISBN: 978-93-5128-143-6
Price: ₹ 650/-

First Published 2016

Published by

Kalpaz Publications
C-30, Satyawati Nagar,
Delhi - 110052
E-mail: kalpaz@hotmail.com Ph.: 9212142040
Printed at : G. Print Process, Delhi

Cataloging in Publication Data--DK

Courtesy: D.K. Agencies (P) Ltd. <docinfo@dkagencies.com>

Mehta, Pallavi, author.

Ageing, nutrition and health / Pallavi M. Mehta, Komal B. Chauhan.
pages cm
Study conducted in India.
Includes bibliographical references.
ISBN 9789351281436

1. Older people--Home care--India. 2. Caregivers--India. 3. Older people--Nutrition--India. 4. Older people--Health and hygiene--India. I. Chauhan, Komal, author. II. Title.

HV1484.I4M44 2015 DDC 362.60954 23

Contents

Foreword

Population aging is a Global phenomenon. As per World Bank's projections, by 2045 the number of adults above the age of 60 will surpass the number of children below the age of 15 years - a demographic tectonic shift .

In India, the number of older persons' population is likely to be more than 70 Million by 2025 A.D. This drastic rise in the number is going to pose many challenges to India, as India has already attained a significant rise in Life Expectancy .

Nowadays older persons do not enjoy same respectful status in Society compared to a few decades back, but people live longer and healthier lives and are capable of substantial contribution to society ; at the same time these elderly are vulnerable to exclusions, marginalisation and discrimination by family and society . Malnutrition and Poor Health of elderly is a reality in Developed as well as Developing countries.

Inadequate Data Base on Health of Local Elderly Population and their Living Conditions, Insufficiency of Funds and Improper Health Care Programme are major contributing factors undermining Healthy Ageing in India.

In this context this book "Ageing, Nutrition and Health" seems to be a sincere effort as it touches on important issues relevant to our elderly and their care givers. I am sure the book will serve as useful reading and reference material to the Academicians, Students, Researchers as also General Public interested in Geriatrics or responsible for well being of elderly at home or as professionals.

In the First Two Chapters the Scenario of Health, Nutrition and Disease Profiles of elderly are shown in different settings, giving good idea about conditions in which they live.

Secrets of Higher Longevity is highlighted in next Chapter based on studies on elderly living beyond the age of 85 to more than 100 years.

Mental Health is of vital importance and is greatly affected by Nutrition and other environmental factors .This has been discussed well particularly in relation to Cognitive Functions, Depression and Dementia in Chapter IV.

In Chapter V and VI Dietary Guidelines for older people and Specially Formulated and Designed Geriatric Foods and Diets have been discussed. This may be useful to all adult population including Elderly, their Care Givers and Elderly to be.

Other important aspects of Care Giving –which is a major emerging need of today's elderly - are also discussed in Chapter VII.

Appendices give useful information relevant to Nutrition and Health Issues for Geriatric group.

I wish to congratulate the Authors for their creation which is for a very good and noble cause of elevating the Health and Nutritional status of Elderly in India and also contributes to existing knowledge about relevant aspects of Gerontology. I am hopeful that with efforts such as these, we will find a way to Power aging in near future.

In the end, I would like to quote the favourite prayer of Swami Vivekanand, which has been chanted by millions of people in India from last five thousand years –

सर्वे भवन्तु सुखिनः
सर्वे सन्तु निरामयाः।
सर्वे भद्राणि पश्यन्तु
मा कश्चिद् दुःखभाग् भवेत्॥

"Let all be Happy, Let all be Healthy. Let all attain Greatness, Let none get misery"

Swami Nikhilanandaji,
Ram Krishna Mission, Vadodara, India

Preface

"Grow old with me, for the best is yet to be"

—Robert Browny

Ageing is a multidimensional phenomenon which concerns all the countries of the world. Presently, India is home to one out of every ten senior citizens of the world. Therefore, the rapid growth in the number of older population presents issues which have hardly been perceived so far. These issues need to be addressed if social and economic development is to proceed effectively. However, we still have the "window of opportunity" to look into current issues concerning diet, disease and nutrition profile of present geriatric population and subsequently generate factual information which can help our national policy planners to design strategies for geriatric welfare in time before "Age quake" happens in terms of dramatic increase in population aged 80 yrs.

Elderly support ratio expressed as the number of working age people ages 15 to 64 divided by the number of persons 65 or older, in India was 13 in 2010 which would decrease to 5 in 2050. This decline is a matter of concern in the economic security of the elderly in India.

There are many centenarians or elderly above 90 years living perfectly healthy life. The secret behind this can be unveiled by studies focused on their life style.

Cognitive ageing is one of the fearful aspects as it is a major burden for the society because of its profound influences on independence and quality of life.

Usually the deterioration of health will begin particularly after the age of 75 yrs which therefore will cause the elderly suffering long standing illness disability or infirmity. The ageing population with increased morbidity may realise care both from informal and formal sectors.

Most of the caregivers whether home bound, professionally paid or from institutions often do not possess adequate knowledge about old age related problems, care and elements of positive health.

Medical science has advanced but each drug that is administered to a patient has its own effects. Geriatric group is often more vulnerable to such effects. Caregivers need to have adequate knowledge about drugs and their adverse reactions in elderly.

Knowledge about relationship of diet with ageing and disease is equally oriented as geriatric medicine. Quality of geriatric care can be greatly improved with enrichment of knowledge and training.

There is no dearth of foods for young children or for specific disease condition. However, special geriatric foods still do not appear in the market even today. Awareness regarding national Policies and plans is totally or partially absent in majority of geriatric population.

This book is therefore a sincere effort which can serve as useful guide to the geriatric caregivers, professionals in the field of geriatrics, students and teachers pursuing geriatric research and common man who is caregiver or elderly to be.

The book includes following chapters;

1. **Ageing population: Socio demographic profile:** This chapter summarises the findings of the studies carried out on urban, rural and tribal elderly population in and around Vadodara.

2. **Old Age homes and Elderly:** The chapter focuses on living conditions of institutionalised elderly and reports in depth studies conducted in Gujarat. Recommendations have been derived.
3. **Stepping the ladder of ageing:** morbidity profile, studies concerning diets of elderly (90+), physical activity profile and other factors responsible for ageing have been discussed and supported by relevant studies.
4. **Mental health and ageing:** This chapter deals with mainly two major problems of mental health namely depression and dementia. Data of some selected studies and studies conducted locally on geriatric population have been presented at appropriate places while highlighting the relationship between cognitive functions and other factors.
5. **Guidelines for diet and nutritional disorders of elderly:** In this chapter, information regarding diet of elderly and guidelines on various nutritional disorders have been given.
6. **Foods for geriatric feeding:** This is a very important chapter which highlights the need for designer foods or elderly problems leading to food inadequacy and intervention to solve these problems, relevant studies carried out by authors and feeding in special condition alongwith a list of food items suggested for geriatric group.
7. **Caregiving: Emerging need of elderly today:** The chapter includes information on the reasons for increasing need of caregiving facilities, problems of caregiving, home caregivers, self-caregiver and professional self-caregivers along with relevant studies.
8. **Some useful information**
9. **Remarks and recommendations:** These are based on authors experience in the field of gerontology and geriatrics and studies conducted by their research team on various issues of ageing.

10. **Appendices:** Include very useful information for geriatric group covering various aspects.

Issues explored in this book and supported by studies mentioned in the chapters are of great relevance and importance for ageing individuals and policy makers for elderly in India. However, the conclusions drawn and opinions expressed are of the authors and are published here as a contribution to the current debate in progressing nations on the issues to be considered in relation to ageing society.

We are sure that the book will serve as useful reading to the academicians, politicians and common public as well. If this be so, our contribution to geriatric community is already rewarded.

Pallavi M. Mehta
Komal B. Chauhan

Acknowledgement

The authors wish to express their deep sense of gratitude to members of Geriatric Research Team of Department of Foods and Nutrition, Faculty of Family and Community Sciences, The M.S. University, Vadodara, India for their immense contribution in executing the Research Studies covered in this book.

We are thankful to Dr. D.V. Bala, Professor and Head, Department of Community Medicine, Smt. N.H.L. Municipal Medical College Ahmedabad for taking keen interest in providing information on important aspects of Geriatrics as well as National Policies on Elderly.

Our profound thanks are also due to our dear students who were involved in the Field Research and Data Collection in Local area and Institutions.

We are extremely grateful to Pujya Swami Nikhileshwaranandji of Ram Krishna Mission Vadodara, India; for writing the Foreword of this book and for blessing us.

We also wish to acknowledge help rendered by Ms Meenakshi Sutaria in typing of the manuscript.

Finally, we thank Kalpaz Publications, New Delhi for publishing the book.

Pallavi M Mehta
Komal B. Chauhan

1

Our Elderly: Situational Analysis of Demography, Diet and Health Profile

"Add life to your years and not years to your life"

—Unknown

Demographic transition in the world has been characterised by the considerable increase in the absolute and relative numbers of elderly people. This has been especially true in the case of developing countries like India, where ageing is occurring more rapidly due to the decline in fertility rates combined by increase in life expectancy of people achieved through medical interventions. About 60 per cent of the elderly live in the developing world, and this will rise to 70 per cent by 2010. Most of this growth will take place in developing countries and over half of it will be in Asia, namely India and China (Rajan et. al., 1999).

According to the 2001 Census of India, life expectancy was 61.9 years for men and 63.1 years for women and is still increasing. This has led to a significant increase in the population of elderly individuals.

Table given below shows number, proportion and sex ratio of the Indian elderly from the year 2001 to 2051.

Table I: Number, proportion and sex ratio of Indian elderly 2001-2051

	2001	*2011**	*2021**	*2031**	*2041**	*2051**
60 and above						
Numbers in million	77	96	133	179	336	301
Percentage to the total population	7.5	8.2	9.9	11.9	14.5	17.3
Sex ratio (males per 1000 females)	1028	1034	1004	964	1008	1007
70 and above						
Numbers in million	29	36	51	73	98	132
Percentage to the total population	2.9	3.1	3.8	4.8	6	7.6
Sex ratio (males per 1000 females)	991	966	970	930	891	954
80 and above						
Numbers in million	8	9	11	16	23	32
Percentage to the total population	0.5	0.7	0.8	1	1.4	1.8
Sex ratio (males per 1000 females)	1051	884	866	843	774	732

Source: Census Survey, 2001
*Projected Figures

The highest proportion of elderly among states and union territories are located in Kerala (10.5 per cent) and lowest proportion was found in Dadra & Nagar Haveli (4.0 per cent). Life expectancy is 61.9 years for men and 63.1 years for women and is still increasing. This has led to a significant increase in the population of elderly individuals.

Rural population is on increase. According to Census 2001, 80 per cent of the elderly populations live in rural areas. The rural elderly are older than the urban elderly, but have little access to tertiary care services. In the rural areas 7.8 per cent of the women are elderly. Census 2001 show that sex ratios favour females and indicates that there are more women than men aged 60 years.

As shown in Table II, Gujarat elderly population is also high with 6.9 per cent of the total population being elderly (age more than 60 years). From this 6.9 per cent of elderly population 66.3 per cent elderly population lives in rural areas. Majority (53.8 per cent) of the rural elderly who reside in Gujarat are females (Census, 2001).

Table III shows distribution of elderly population according to residence and sex. At Vadodara district level, 7 per cent of total population are elderly. Of this, 57.4 per cent of the elderly live in rural areas of which 53.1 per cent are females (Census, 2001). This shows that more number of elderly live in rural areas and females comprise of more than half of this population.

Lifestyle Factors

Life style of a person right from the childhood till death will decide upon the wellbeing at every phase of life.

An overview of the longitudinal survey in Europe on nutrition and the elderly, which was designed to assess differences in dietary and lifestyle factors among elderly Europeans, and to identify the factors that contribute to healthy ageing revealed that, the smoking prevalence among women was generally low. A healthy lifestyle was related to stable self-perceived health, a delay in functional dependence, and mortality. Inactivity and smoking increased mortality risk. The study showed that a healthy lifestyle at older ages is related to a delay in the deterioration of health status and a reduced mortality risk (Lisette et al., 2004).

With the purpose of studying the health-promoting lifestyle behaviours of 102 community-dwelling rural women aged 65 years and older and to determine the extent to which personal influences (demographics, definition of health, and perceived health status) and contextual influences (sources of health information and provider counseling) explain health-promoting lifestyle behaviours. Pullen et al. (2001) found that rural elderly women scored highest on frequency

Table II: Elderly Population of Gujarat by Residence and Sex

Age Group	*Total*			*Rural*			*Urban*		
	Persons	*Males*	*Females*	*Persons*	*Males*	*Females*	*Persons*	*Males*	*Females*
60-64	1297301	625662	671639	862383	412250	450133	434918	213412	221506
65-69	892465	418028	474437	585605	271612	313993	306860	146416	160444
70-74	650698	303145	347553	433701	201498	232203	216997	101647	115350
75-79	284362	126396	157966	184383	80871	103512	99979	45525	54454
80+	374237	155243	218994	252879	106029	146850	121358	49214	72144
Total	3499063	1628474	1870589	2318951	1072260	1246691	1180112	556214	623898

Source: Census Survey, 2001

Table III: Elderly Population of Vadodara District by Residence and Sex

Age Group	*Total*			*Rural*			*Urban*		
	Persons	*Males*	*Females*	*Persons*	*Males*	*Females*	*Persons*	*Males*	*Females*
60-64	98576	48055	50521	57552	27260	30292	41024	20795	20229
65-69	68290	32773	35517	39334	18566	20768	28956	14207	14749
70-74	45853	21469	24384	26694	12368	14326	19159	9101	10058
75-79	20595	9358	11237	10732	4948	5784	9863	4410	5453
80+	23420	10294	13126	13092	5920	7172	10328	4374	5954
Total	256734	121949	134785	147404	69062	78342	109330	52887	56443

of nutrition behaviours and lowest on frequency of physical activity behaviours. Multiple regression analyses revealed that younger age, living with other(s), defining health as wellness, better perceived mental health, more sources of health information and provider counseling were significantly associated with health-promoting lifestyle behaviours.

When determinants of leisure time physical activity (LTPA) in rural (n=1242) and urban (n=1096) middle aged and older women were studied. Sara Wilcox et al. (2000) found that rural women, and less educated women, were more sedentary than urban women. Rural women reported more personal barriers to LTPA, cited caregiving duties as their top barrier (compared with lack of time for urban women), and had greater body mass indices. Rural elderly women were less likely to report sidewalks, streetlights, high crime, and access to facilities. Women with higher levels of baseline physical activity were less likely to develop cognitive decline (Yaffeet et al., 2001; Weuve et al., 2004).

Ringsberg et al. (2001) studied the impact of long-term moderate physical activity on functional performance, bone mineral density and fracture incidence in rural elderly women and concluded that elderly women, who continue with moderate exercise programmes over many years, sustain fewer fractures and have better muscle strength, balance, gait and health ratings than women in general.

Alcohol and substance abuse among the elderly is a hidden national epidemic. Alcohol use disorders in elderly people are common and associated with considerable morbidity. They are associated with notable impairments in physical, social, psychological, and cognitive health. The problem once was thought largely to affect males, but that assumption is changing. (Connell et al., 2003). The prevalence of smoking bidi/cigarette/hukka, tobacco chewing and alcohol drinking was much higher in rural areas than in urban areas. One -fifth of them chew pan masala or tobacco in rural areas whereas 13 per cent chew the same in urban areas. Alcohol drinking is higher in rural areas than in urban areas (Swain, 2004).

A community level descriptive study by Kumari (2001) was carried out in Sreekaryampanchaya, Kerala on 200 rural elderly females and found that although females have less addiction, rural 51.57 per cent of females were pan chewers.

Devi (2005) highlighted the general problems faced by the aged Indian women. She reported that feeling of insecurity is prevalent in widows and in those whose children are not living with them. There is lack of purpose in life of a women whose life had been centered on that of husband who dies. Indian elderly women are also at risk of facing psychosomatic syndromes, where loneliness, resentment and depression can lead to physical symptoms and may develope chronic illnesses like pains and aches, breathlessness etc.

Kohli et al. (2006) carried out a study on 160 elderly of Punjab, using random sampling technique and found that majority of rural elderly females were widows (88.75 per cent) which increases the problem magnitude as the aged who lost the spouse are often forced to give up independent household, move with children or relative, give up claim on property and become dependent due to disintegrating system, low income, inadequate accommodation, ill health, loneliness and negligence. Majority of the rural females (82.50 per cent) were found to be illiterates, thus preventing them from being self sufficient. Hence 70 per cent had financial problems and did not have sufficient amount to spend as and when required.

Living conditions do affect ageing. Radkar and Kaulagekar (2006) used the data of National Family Health Survey-2 and gave an overview of living conditions of elderly in India. It was reported that urban elderly enjoy the comforts of day-to-day life whereas their rural counterparts are deprived of basic needs like water, toilet and electricity, which also indicates vulnerability of rural elderly. More number of the subjects was found to be widow and three per cent of them were staying alone, with no one to look after.

Dhar, H. (2001) reports that cultural and social forces affect elderly's personal health attribute and their sick propensity. Involvements in religious activities were associated with positive mental and physical health. Lack of social support was associated with risk of mortality, supportive relationships was associated with lower illness rates, faster recovery rates and higher levels of health care behaviour.

Yadav et al. (2003) carried out a study on 96 Indian elderly and reported that high prevalence of dental problems (> 89 per cent) in the elderly subjects prevented them from enjoying their meals and was found to be the major factor for reported reduction in dietary intake with advancement of age.

Morbidity is also a factor which affects ageing. In a case control study, Singh et al. (2003) studied 730 individuals belonging to different age groups and was found that cataract prevalence increased significantly with increasing age, particularly for individuals older than 70 years ($p<0.001$).

Diet and morbidity profile: Situational analysis

Nutrition is viewed traditionally as the specific dietary requirements of different age groups, without exploring diet in the context of a life-long contributory factor to well-being.

Many studies conducted by author on elderly have shown that the energy, protein, iron, calcium, β-carotene, vit-C and fiber intake were significantly less than the RDA (Shah and Mehta, 1995; Shringarpure and Mehta, 2004; Panchal et al., 2005; Chauhan and Mehta, 2007).

A study by Chhabra and Mehta (2001) on 80 urban elderly in Baroda reported that nutrient intake of edentulous elderly through routine diet was insufficient and dentures resulted in significant improvement in nutritional status of elderly men.

Lee and Frongillo (2001) examined the consequences associated with food insecurity for the nutritional and health status of the elderly in the United States and reported that food-insecure elderly were likely to have lower nutrient intake, skin fold thickness, self-reported health status and higher nutritional risk. Regardless of food in security status, older people consumed less than the recommended dietary allowance for eight nutrients. Food-insecure elderly persons had significantly lower intake of energy, protein, carbohydrate, saturated fat, niacin, riboflavin, vitamins B-6 and B-12, magnesium, iron and zinc, as well as lower skinfold thickness and concluded that food-insecure elderly persons have poorer dietary intake, nutritional status and health status than do food-secure elderly persons. According to WHO national household survey in former Yugoslav Republic of Macedonia (1999), the mean frequency of food consumption is lower in households which consist only of elderly people.

Consumption of fruits and vegetables by elderly people (n = 369) living in Nottingham, England, was analysed in relation to whether or not they were eating five portions a day. Those respondents who were older and less educated ate fewer vegetables and those respondents who had a lower income or social grade ate less fruit (Donkin et al. 2002).

Morbidity has been defined as "any departure, subjective or objective, from a state of physiological well-being. The term is used equivalent to such terms as sickness, illness disability WHO expert committee on Health Statistics noted on its 6th report that morbidity could be measured in terms of 3 units.

(i) Persons who were ill.

(ii) The illnesses (provides number of spells of illness) that these persons experienced.

(iii) The duration (days, weeks etc.) of these illnesses.

The Indian attitude that illness is a part of old age is very much deep rooted. There is inadequate appreciation of the need for geriatric health care practices in India. Ranking of various, social, economic and psychological problems of respondents revealed 'Health Problems' as the major problem and ranked first among the respondents from India. 'Financial difficulties' stood out as the fourth problem among the respondents from India. This indirectly affects the morbidity pattern of elderly (Ramachandran and Radhika, 2006). A community based study by Shah et al. (2004) studied a total of 1240 (716 urban and 524 rural) elderly people found that 60 per cent were dissatisfied with their function of mastication because of loss of teeth and lack of dentures. The level of edentulousness was found to be high, more so in rural than in urban people and more so in advancing age. Only <50 per cent of those needing complete dentures and <13 per cent of those needing partial dentures were wearing dentures. The denture needs of the rural elderly were higher than those of the urban elderly. Vegetarians had a higher level of edentulousness compared with non-vegetarians. The BMI was not correlated with level of edentulousness.

Ramachandran and Radhika (2006) reported that visual problem, difficulty in walking, heart problem, diabetes mellitus, rheumatoid arthritis, osteoporosis, hypertension, fatigue and other health problems were high among the respondents from India.

Joshi et al. (2006) collected comprehensive data on health and elderly from four different income groups of elderly population (n=163). The result shows that hypertension and diabetes mellitus are prevalent disorders of middle class population, while anemia was most common in lower strata.

Rajan et al. (2005) studied elderly women (n=5013) and disclosed that 40 per cent of the elderly suffer from at least one disability, incidence being higher among females compared to males.

According to WHO (2002), over a lifetime, women lose about 40 per cent of their skeletal calcium, approximately one half in the first five years after menopause and the remainder at a slower rate thereafter. A longitudinal population-based study by Jones et al. (1994), documents the incidence of all symptomatic fractures from 1989 to 1992 in an elderly (n = 271). The study reported that residual lifetime fracture risk in a person aged 60 years with average life expectancy was 29 per cent for males and 56 per cent for females. Lund et al. (2000) studied 70-95 years old women and men (n = 911) and reported that women aged 70-74 years with continuously low contact frequency showed an increased mortality compared to women constantly experiencing high contact frequency. Among women aged 75 + years living alone was a significant predictor of mortality, when compared to women continuously living with somebody. And the associations seemed stronger among women than men. Authors studies on older adults (70+ to 104 years) have been reported elsewhere in this book.

Amongst the studied 4800 rural population, 3.36 per cent of elderly was found to be blind, with cataract being the single most important cause. (Vijaya et al., 2005). There are associations with accessing health care, family support and financial needs.

A study by Wanless (2001) on 8,468 elderly rural-urban women (65+ years) of Canada reported that 88.1 per cent had any chronic condition, 47.4 per cent had arthritis, 41.8 per cent had high blood pressure, 11.2 per cent had diabetes and 17.6 per cent had heart disease. It was concluded that elderly women in rural areas were more likely to have any chronic condition, high blood pressure, diabetes and heart disease.

The study conducted in the urban and rural areas Chandigarh on 362 elderly (>65 years) by Sharma et al. (2007) revealed that the overall prevalence of osteo-arthritis was 56.6 per cent, in rural it was 32.6 per cent and in urban it was 66.6 percent and the prevalence was more in females compared to that of males.

A study conducted by authors (Mehta et al., 2008) on 130 female elderly belonging to rural settings of Vadodara district of Gujarat state, India, with respect to diet, health and disease profile with relation to socio-demographic status showed interesting results when compared to their urban counterparts.

Following conclusions were drawn from the findings of Vadodara urban and rural studies:

- There were distinct differences in diet, nutrition and disease profile of rural elderly women in comparison to ones reported by studies on urban elderly women.
- Age and income level appear to be important determinants of health
- Widowhood seems to be a common feature in rural women which in turn results in increased burden of social, economic and healthcare services for this underprivileged section of the society
- Anaemic status and grossly inadequate nutrient intake are the major contributors of ill health in rural elderly female population
- Mental health status of rural poor elderly has been found to be inferior with regard to depression status and cognitive functions
- This suggests further need for interventions like counselling and pharmaceutical management of mental illness

There is very scanty literature available on the tribal elderly. Authors attempted to study 100 elderly males and females residing in tribal setting in local Vadodara district, Gujarat state, India (Mehta and co workers, 2011). The data on nutrition, diet and health profile of these tribal elderly showed a very different picture.

Following are the key observations of this research:

- Tribal population showed a very high prevalence of illiteracy and widowhood in female elderly.

- Bidi and Gutka consumption were common in elderly population. There was high prevalence of oral cavity problems in tribal elderly.
- Diet of tribal elderly was deficient in all nutrients. There was a simple meal pattern in their daily diet.
- Prevalence of anaemia and underweight were prominent observations.
- There was hardly any inclusion of dairy products and vegetables in their diet.
- Oral cavity and locomotor problems ranked highest followed by Gastro-intestinal tract problems in these elderly.
- There was deterioration of mental health profile with age.
- Depression was highly prevalent in tribal elderly females.

Thus, situational analysis of urban, rural and tribal elderly show very distinct scenario in the Indian context. Since elderly form a very large segment of total population, it has been a worthwhile attempt to explore the conditions under which our elderly live, as such data may act as useful inputs for policy makers.

References

Census India (2001), Office of the Registrar General and Census Commissioner, India available at:http://www.censusindia.gov.in

Chhabra S and Mehta P, 2001, A study on nutritional status, diet and disease profile of edentulous elderly subjects (with and without denture treatment) M.Sc. Dissertation (unpublished), Dept. of Foods and Nutrition, The M.S. University, Baroda, India.

Connell H, Chin A, Cunningham C, Lawlor B and Norma C, (2003) Alcohol use disorders in elderly people-redefining an age old problem in old age, BMJ; 327(7416): 664-667.

Devi P (2005) Ageing and Gerontology in the context of Women in India, Indian Journal of Gerontology; Vol. 19, No. 3, pp. 350-355.

Dhar H (2001), Gender, ageing, health and society, J Assoc Physicians India.; Vol. 49 : 1012-20.

Donkin A, Johnson A, Lilley J, Morgan K, Neale R, Page R and Silburn R (2002), Gender and Living Alone as Determinants of Fruit and Vegetable Consumption among the Elderly Living at Home in Urban Nottingham Science Direct; 30 (1): 39-51.

Haveman-Nies A, Groot L, Staveren W (2003), Dietary quality, lifestyle factors and healthy ageing in Europe: the SENECA study, Age and Ageing; 32: 427-434.

Kohli N, Dhillon M, Sidhu M and Singh H (2006), Analytical study of economic problems faced by the elderly single and suggestions to improve these problems, Indian Journal of Gerontology; 20(4): 417-430.

Lee J and Frongillo E (2001), Nutritional and Health Consequences Are Associated with Food Insecurity among U.S. Elderly Persons, Journal of Nutrition; 131: 1503-1509.

Mehta P, Chauhan K, Patel K and Singh N (2008) Assessment of diet, nutrition and disease profile of elderly females and males residing in rural setting of Vadodara, unpublished masters dissertation, Department of Foods and Nutrition, The M.S. University of Baroda, Vadodara, Gujarat.

Mehta P, Chauhan K, Desai P and Mahendra M (2011) Situational analysis of nutrition, diet and health profile of tribal elderly males and females of selected villages in sankhedataluka of Vadodara, unpublished masters dissertation, Department of Foods and Nutrition, The M.S. University of Baroda, Vadodara, Gujarat.

Panchal P and Mehta P (2000), A study on Nutrition, Diet and Disease profile of elderly patients with dental problem M.Sc. Dissertation (unpublished), Dept. of Foods and Nutrition, The M.S. University, Baroda, India.

Patel D and Mehta P (1999), A study on lifestyle factors, nutritional status and Dietary profile of women and men in relation to osteoporotic fractures: NHE program as a strategy for prevention (age 50 years onwards) M.Sc. Dissertation (unpublished), Dept. of Foods and Nutrition, The M.S. University, Baroda, India.

Pullen, Carol E, Walker, Noble S, Fiandt, Kathryn (2001), Determinants of Health-Promoting Lifestyle Behaviors in Rural Older Women, Family and Community Health; 24(2):49-72.

Radkar A and Kaulagekar A (2006), Problems of Elderly Women in India and Japan, Indian Journal of Gerontology; 20(3): 250-263.

Ringsberg K, Gardsell P, Johnell O, Josefsson P and Obrant K (2001), The Impact of Long-Term Moderate Physical Activity on Functional Performance, Bone Mineral Density and Fracture Incidence in Elderly Women, Gerontology; 47:15-20.

Shah N, Parkash H and Sunderam K (2004), Edentulousness, denture wear and denture needs of Indian elderly - a community-based study, Journal of Oral Rehabilitation; 31(5): 467-476.

Sharma M, Swami H, Bhatia V, Verma A, Bhatia S, Kaur G (2007), An Epidemiological Study of Correlates of Osteo-Arthritis in Geriatric Population of UT Chandigarh, Indian Journal of Community Medicine; 32(1).

Singh M, Murthy G and Venkatraman R (2003), Risk factors of senile cataract among elderly persons aged 50 years and above in rural areas of wardha in maharashtra Indian Journal of Gerontology; 17(3 and 4): 325-334.

Swain P and Raj T (2003), Demography of Ageing in India: State and District level Analysis, Indian Journal of Gerontology; 19(3): 327-342.

Swain P (2004), Socio-Demographic and health of Widows in India, National Institute of Health and Family Welfare, available at: http://www.nihfw.nic.in/asp/ResearchStudies.asp

United Nations Population Division (1998), World Population Prospects: The 2002 Revision available at: http://www.un.org/esa/population/publications/wpp2002/WPP2002-HIGHLIGHTSrev1.PDF

Weuve J, Kang J, Manson J, Breteler M, Grodstein. F (2003), Physical Activity, Including Walking, and Cognitive Function in Older Women, The journal of American medical association; 292(12): 1454-1461.

WHO (2002), Active Ageing: A Policy Framework, WHO, Spain

WHO (2002), Keep Fit For Life- Meeting the Nutritional Needs of Older persons WHO; Tufts University, School of Nutrition and Policy.

Yadav R, Prakash S and Kumar P (2003), Dietary habits, nutritional status and levels of serum vitamine in healthy older adults in India, Indian Journal of Gerontology; 17(3 and 4): 375-379.

Yaffe K, Barnes D, Nevitt M, Li-Yung Lui, Covinsky K (2001), A Prospective Study of Physical Activity and Cognitive Decline in Elderly Women, Arch Intern Med; 161: 1703-1708.

2

Our Old Age Homes and Elderly

"Trees grow stronger over the years, rivers wider. Likewise, with age, human beings gain immeasurable depth and breadth of experience and wisdom. That is why older persons should be not only respected and revered, they should be utilised as the rich resource to society that they are":

–United Nations Secretary General Kofi Annan.

India is presently undergoing demographic transition. Due to change in recent demographic trend, population of elderly in India is on rise. This population ageing phenomenon in our country has great implications on the health and social welfare systems. India, like many traditional societies today faces a unique situation in providing care for its elderly because of fast diminishing old age support and structures. Therefore old age homes are felt as a necessity in the present day scenario as the younger generation is having problems in coping up with special needs of the elderly and required resources for the special care. Though there is recent increase in the number of old age homes, whether it is satisfactory situation under which elderly live in old age homes is questionable. There is dearth of information on living conditions of institutionalised elderly within the country. In this chapter attempt has been made to present available information with more focus on Gujarat where in depth studies were carried out recently.

As per report published in Help Age India, 1998, there are 728 old age homes in India today. Some information is available only about 547 homes. Out of these, 325 homes are free of cost while 95 old age homes are on pay and stay basis and 11 homes have no information.

A total of 278 old age homes all over the country are available for sick and 101 homes are exclusively for women. Kerala has 124 old age homes which is maximum as compared to any state.

A study conducted in 2008 has reported major reasons for staying at old age homes as "neglected and living alone", physical insecurity", neglect after decreased income contribution", "lower medical and living cost", "physical and verbal abuse by family", "neglect by family due to high health care cost", "poverty" and others (Goel and Gupta, 2008).

Author conducted its first study simultaneously on two old age homes of Vadodara (Mehta and Limaye, 1999) which showed lot of differences between both the homes in terms of living arrangement and food pattern. Inclusion of all food groups, facilities like lift, room service on payment basis and recreational activities time to time found in Jalaram Vanprashthashram created better environment to live as compared to Premdas Jalaram Vridhashram.

A study on old age home in Chandigarh (Gurjeet, 2010) reported economic, social and adjustment reasons for shifting to old age homes. The study also revealed that residents not only faced problems related to room sharing, cleanliness and inadequate food but also majority faced lack of medical facilities, recreational facilities and harsh and impolite staff behaviour.

Some of the screening methods can only be administered by trained clinicians. Biochemical markers are time consuming and expensive to use in home situations, and the criteria for their interpretation in old age are unclear.

Old Age Homes in Gujarat

Attempts have been made to list the old age homes from the available information (refer appendix 5). A detailed study was conducted on different old age homes and their inmates situated in four major cities of Gujarat state. A total of twelve institutions, three from each city were selected from Vadodara, Ahmedabad, Surat and Rajkot.

(A) Infrastructure Facilities

Data on infrastructure facilities are shown in the table below:

Table I: Percentage of institutes showing various infrastructure facilities (n = 12)

Sr. No.	*Facility*	*Present (%)*	*Absent (%)*
1	Sitting room/lounge	75 (9)	25 (3)
2	Compound	66.67 (8)	33.33 (4)
3	Kitchen	100 (12)	0 (0)
4	Dining hall	83.33 (10)	16.67 (2)
5	Temple/Prayer room	91.67 (11)	8.33 (1)
6	Recreation room (TV, games, exercise, computer)	75 (9)	25 (3)
7	Library	58.33 (7)	41.67 (5)
8	Physiotherapy centre	41.67 (5)	58.33 (7)
9	Railing	83.33 (10)	16.67 (2)
10	Swings	83.33 (10)	16.67 (2)
11	Lift (institutions having more than ground floor, n=8)	50 (4)	50 (4)

All the institutions had kitchen facilities. Fifty per cent institutions had facility of library, physiotherapy centre and lift. Details of other special facilities provided to the inmates are shown in the table II.

Table II: Percentage of institutes providing various facility/services to the inmates (n=12)

Sr. No.	*Facility*	*Yes (%)*	*No (%)*
1.	Transport (bus, van, bus pass, etc)	50 (6)	50 (6)
2.	Security	83.33 (10)	16.67 (2)
3.	Adequate water supply	100 (12)	0 (0)
4.	Wheelchair/walking sticks	83.33 (10)	16.66 (2)
5.	Individual toilet/bathroom	75 (9)	25(3)
6.	Individual attendant for special needs	41.67(5)	58.33(7)
7.	Call for help (bell, telephone)	41.67(5)	58.33(7)
8.	Permission to meet family & friends	91.67(11)	8.33 (1)
9.	Recreational trips	75 (9)	25 (3)
	Frequency (n=9)		
	a) ≤ 2/ year	33.33(3)	
	b) ≥ 3/year	66.67 (6)	
10.	Promoting hobbies	58.33(7)	41.67(5)
11.	Religious activities	83.33 (10)	16.67(2)

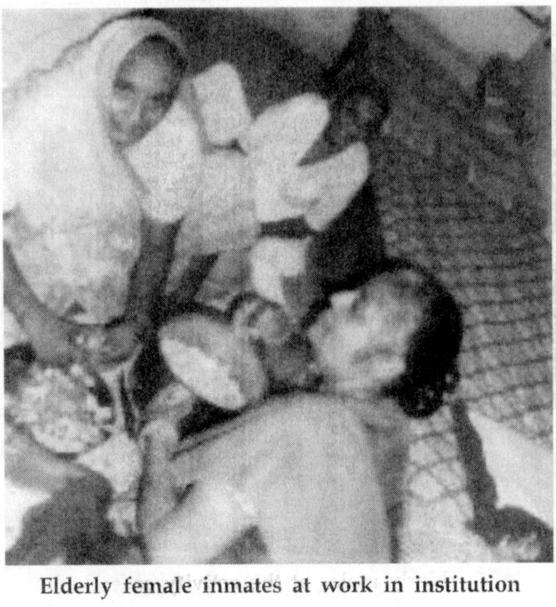

Elderly female inmates at work in institution

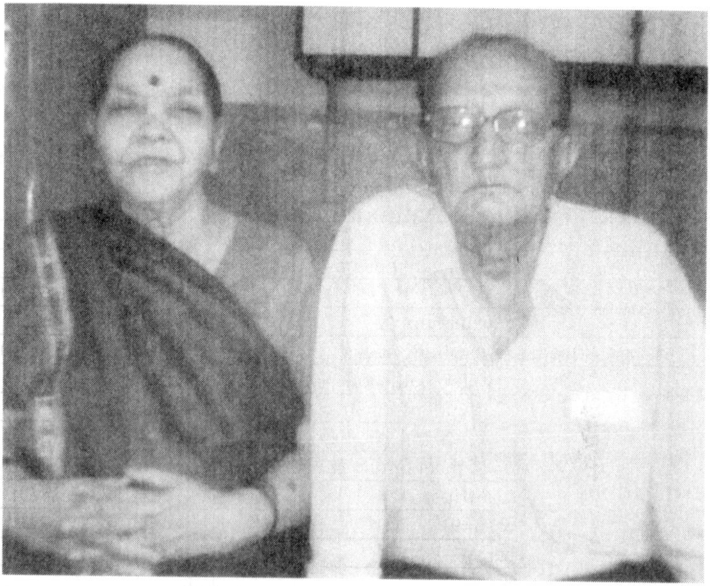

Elderly couple in an institution

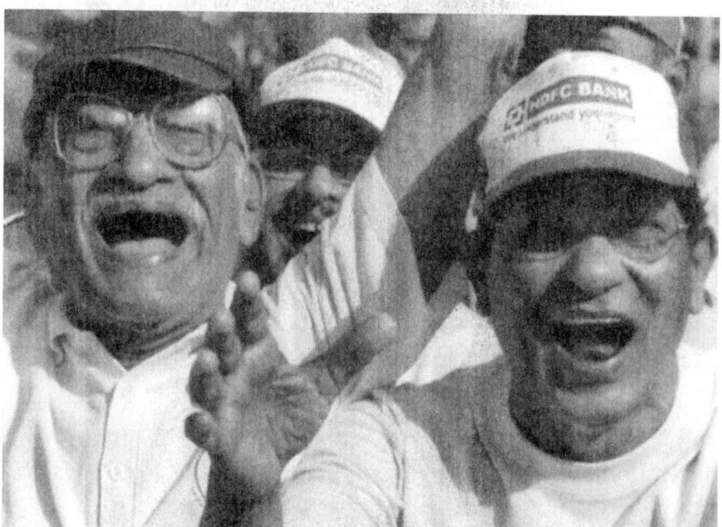

Elderly males at the activity center

Seventy-five per cent institutes provided first aid facility and all provided emergency hospital facility. Very few institutions (6-8) had clinics, visits by doctor, post operative care and special diets for critically ill patients.

(B) Food Related Practices

In all institutions unlimited food was provided. Seven institutes provided less than 3 meals per day. Majority served food at right temperature and provided milk and milk products.

Nearly half of the institutes' had good ambience in dining hall and personal hygiene of the kitchen staff was well observed in these institutions. Majority of the institutions showed good behaviour of the serving staff except in two institutions.

Some good practices regarding general sanitation and hygiene were observed by institutions. Table below reveals data of the institutions following various sanitation and hygiene practices (Table III)

Table III: Percentage of institutes following various sanitation and hygiene practices (n = 12)

Sr.	*Observations*	*Present (%)*	*Absent (%)*
1	Apron	0 (0)	100 (0)
2	Head gear	0 (0)	100 (0)
3	Clean hands	83.33 (8)	16.67 (2)
4	Trimmed nails	41.67(5)	58.33(7)
5	Washing of vegetables before	100 (12)	0 (0)
6	Use of clean utensils	100 (12)	0 (0)
7	Cleaning of cooking area	100 (12)	0 (0)
8	Garbage disposal	100 (12)	0 (0)

Meal pattern differed in all the institutions though all institutions provided lunch and dinner. Table IV shows the percentage of institutes showing the meal pattern.

Table IV: Percentage of institution showing the meal pattern (n=12)

Sr.	Meal	Yes (%)	No (%)
1	Breakfast	50 (6)	50 (6)
	(a) Freshly prepared hot snacks (n=6)	33.33 (2)	
	(b) Dry snacks (n=6)	66.67 (4)	
2	Lunch	100 (12)	0 (0)
	(a) Full	100 (12)	
	(b) Half	0 (0)	
3	Dinner	100 (12)	0 (0)
	(a) Full	8.33 (1)	
	(b) Half	50 (6)	
	(c) Variety of food items	41.67 (5)	

(C) Fee Structure

Five institutions provided free stay and services to the inmates whereas rest of the institutes charged fees ranging from Rs. 500 to 1500/-.

All the institutes prohibited addiction for inmates. Use of telephone and going out of the institutes was allowed only after permission in all the institutes.

Situtational Analysis of Inmates of Old Age Homes

In this study of old age homes in Gujarat, elderly females belonging to 60 yrs age and above were selected randomly from different old age homes situated in selected cities of Gujarat state. Baseline data was collected on socio-demographic profile, lifestyle factors, nutritional status, clinical parameters, diet profile, disease profile and mental health status. Data on socio-demographic information of institutionalised female elderly from selected old age homes are presented in table below.

Table V: Socio-demographic information of institutionalised female elderly

Characteristics	*Ahmedabad (N=37)*	*Vadodara (N=38)*	*Rajkot (N=37)*	*Surat (N=37)*	*Total (N=149)*
A) Age (Mean±S.D)	74.14±7.12	73.58±7.08	73.81±9.18	74.49±9.8	74±8.30
B) Marital status					
Married	8.1(3)	28.9(11)	13.5(5)	16.2(6)	16.8(25)
Unmarried	5.4(2)	10.5(4)	10.8(4)	10.8(4)	9.4(14)
Divorced	8.1(3)	5.3(2)	13.5(5)	5.4(2)	8.1(12)
Widow	78.4(29)	55.3(21)	62.2(23)	67.6(25)	65.8(98)
C) Ethnic group					
Gujarati	91.9(34)	86.8(33)	94.6(35)	67.6(25)	85.2(127)
Non- Gujarati	8.1(3)	13.2(5)	5.4(2)	32.4(12)	14.8(22)
D) Stay in old age home					
< 5 years	43.2(16)	50(19)	48.6(18)	75.7(28)	54.4(81)
5- 10 years	32.4(12)	36.8(14)	35.1(13)	18.9(7)	30.9(46)
>10 years	24.3(9)	13.2(5)	16.2(6)	5.4(2)	14.8(22)
E) Education					
Primary	43.2(16)	34.2(13)	54.1(20)	56.8(21)	47(70)
Secondary	10.8(4)	36.8(14)	13.5(5)	16.2(6)	19.5(29)
Graduate	2.7(1)	18.4(7)	5.4(2)	5.4(2)	8.1(12)
Post-graduate	2.7(1)	5.3(2)	0(0)	0(0)	2(3)
Illiterate	40.5(15)	5.3(2)	27(10)	21.6(8)	23.5(35)
F) Family type					
Joint	37.8(14)	34.2(13)	35.1(13)	59.5(22)	41.6(62)
Nuclear	62.2(23)	65.8(25)	64.9(24)	40.5(15)	58.4(87)
G) Source of income					
Savings	21.6(8)	36.8(14)	2.7(1)	29.7(11)	22.8(34)
Pension	2.7(1)	26.3(10)	2.7(1)	5.4(2)	9.4(14)
Dependent on children	24.3(9)	18.4(7)	5.4(2)	27(10)	18.8(28)
Dependent on family members	8.1(3)	18.4(7)	5.4(2)	21.6(8)	13.4(20)
Dependent on institution	43.2(16)	0(0)	83.8(31)	16.2(6)	35.6(53)

Among all the institutions, more than 55 per cent female subjects were widows. Though majority had primary education, almost 1/4th of the population was illiterate and very few had university degree. It was interesting to note that more than half of subjects lived in nuclear family before coming to the old age homes. More than one third of female population was dependent on institutions. Higher number of older females (above 70-80 yrs) required help in daily activities such as walking, climbing stairs, using toilets, dressing up and eating than their younger counter parts (60-70 yrs). It is worth noting that majority of male as well as female subjects were satisfied with the palatability, temperature and variety of food provided in the institution, hygiene at the dining hall, behaviour of the staff members, cleanliness in the room, lighting facilities at night and the overall stay in the institution.

Activity Pattern:

Information on activity pattern showed significant, difference in the mean hours spent for daily activities, religious activities and physical activities between inmates of different cities

Table VI: Mean hours spent per day on different activities by institutionalised female elderly subjects

Type of activity	*Ahmedabad N= 37*	*Vadodara N= 38*	*Rajkot N= 37*	*Surat N= 37*	*Total N=149*	*F value*
Daily activities	5.35±0.71	4.44±0.89	5.18±0.81	4.89±0.73	4.96±0.85	9.42***
Leisure time	2.75±1.38	3.71±1.67	3.10±1.5	3.37±1.53	3.24±1.55	2.62^{NS}
Religious activities	3.35±1.15	2.60±0.88	3.21±1.39	2.4±1.09	2.89±1.2	5.97***
Physical activities	0.43±0.6	0.71±0.75	0	0.38±0.54	0.38±0.6	10.39***
Idle time	5.62±1.8	5.11±2.0	6.11±1.9	5.31±2.3	5.53±2	1.63^{NS}

The inmates of Rajkot were not involved in any type of physical activity. However the later were more involved in the spiritual activities compared to the inmates of the other cities. It was interesting to note that the study also reported higher prevalence of Osteoporosis in elderly with low level of activity. The study also reported that nearly 69 per cent of women were engaged in kitchen activities like vegetable cutting and other kitchen cores.

Below table shows the activity pattern of male subjects.

Table VII: Mean hours spent per day on different activities by institutionalised male elderly subjects

Type of activity	*Vadodara (N=32)*	*Ahmedabad (N=25)*	*Surat (N=24)*	*Rajkot (N=21)*	*Total (N=102)*	*Chi square*
Daily routine activity	4.60±0.74	5.28±0.73	4.91±0.77	5.0±0.83	4.91±0.77	3.62*
Leisure time	3.90±1.64	2.96±1.39	3.33±1.68	3.28±1.34	3.41±1.56	1
Religious activity	2.68±0.89	3.12±1.12	2.37±1.01	2.61±1.11	2.70±1.04	2.23 NS
Exercise	0.57±0.73	0.28±0.54	0.20±0.41	0.0	0.29±0.56	5.42**
Sleep	7.40±1.72	6.36±1.77	7.66±1.78	6.57±1.69	7.03±1.80	3.27*
Idle time	4.90±2.18	5.92±2.01	5.45±2.58	6.71±1.79	5.65±2.24	3.11*

Significance at *P<0.05, **P<0.01

Significant difference in the mean hours spent on activity profile of male elderly in between various institutions was observed especially with regard to exercise and daily routine activities.

Nutritional Status

The study also assessed nutritional status in terms of anthropometric measurement. Table VIII shows mean anthropometric measurements of elderly females inmates of selected old age homes of Gujarat.

Table VIII: Mean anthropometric measurements of institutionalised female elderly subjects

Variable	Ahmedabad (N=37)	Vadodara (N=38)	Rajkot (N=37)	Surat (N=37)	F value
Height (cm)	147.55±6.2	149.94±6.44	152.73±4.5	147.97±8.2	4.89**
Weight (kg)	53.20±10.2	57.53±11.89	61.32±12.75	54.36±15.31	3.05*
BMI (kg/mt²)	24.16±3.73	25.66±5.20	26.24±5.59	24.43±5.87	1.36NS
Waist (cm)	84.46±7.12	91.68±9.14	92.77±11.35	87.04±11.42	5.77***
Hip (cm)	98.49±8.21	103.89±9.07	105.12±12.80	99.03±13.38	3.42*
WHR	0.85±0.05	0.88±0.06	0.88±0.05	0.87±0.06	1.7NS
Demispan(cm)	67.69±5.0	70.25±5.22	90.12±111.72	74.17±6.41	1.34NS

Data on female elderly showed that 1/3rd of them were overweight. However, very few (5 per cent-15 per cent) elderly females were underweight and obese. In case of male subjects as can be seen in table IX, all the subjects had almost similar body mass index/waist to hip ratio, irrespective to different cities.

Table IX: Mean body mass index and waist hip ratio of male elderly subjects

Variable	*Vadodara (N=32)*	*Ahmedabad (N=25)*	*Surat (N=24)*	*Rajkot (N=21)*	*Total (N=102)*	*f-value*
BMI	25.0±3.37	24.38±3.35	23.77±3.35	24.52±4.23	24.46±3.86	0.46 NS
WHR	1.01±0.82	1.0±0.09	1.01±0.65	0.98±0.07	1.06±0.07	0.95 NS

Clinical Signs

Clinical signs and symptoms were checked for iron deficiency anemia and vitamin A deficiency. Following table shows the presence and absence of it in percentage of male and female subjects.

Female elderly inmates showed higher prevalence of anemia whereas vit-A deficiency symptoms were not so common. In case of males 50 per cent subjects had signs of anemia whereas only 13 per cent showed problem of night blindness.

Table X: Percentage of institutionalised in female and male elderly subjects showing clinical signs and symptoms of various deficiency disorders

Signs and symptoms	*Female*		*Male*	
1. Iron Deficiency Anemia	**Present**	**Absent**	**Present**	**Absent**
Pallor- palm	47(70)	53(79)	48(49)	52(53)
Pallor- tongue	47.7(71)	52.3(78)	52.9(54)	47.1(48)
Pallor- conjunctiva	51(76)	49(73)	54.9(56)	45.1(46)
Pallor- nails	61.7(92)	38.3(57)	56.9(58)	43.1(44)
2. Vitamin A Deficiency				
Bitot's spots	0.7(1)	99.3(148)	00(00)	102 (100)
Night blindness	12.8(19)	87.2(130)	12.7(13)	87.3(89)

Diet Profile:

Most of the studies reported so far have shown gross inadequacy of nutrient intake in elderly residing in old age homes. (Bagchi and Puri, 1999, Mehta 1999, 2000, Mehta and Limaye, 1999, Chauhan and Mehta, 2007 and Mehta et al, 2010)

Author's team also studied dietary intake of institutionalised elderly subjects residing in selected old age homes of Gujarat. The data on dietary intake was collected using 24 hour dietary recall. Results are presented in table11.

Table XI (a) and (b): Percentage of individuals showing consumption of different nutrients at various levels of per cent RDA by institutionalised female and male elderly

(a) Female

Nutrients	*RDA**	*%RDA*				
		< 25	*26-50*	*51-75*	*76-100*	*>100*
Energy (K.cal)	1350	0(0)	2.7(4)	23.5(35)	34.2(51)	39.6(59)
Protein (gm)	50	0(0)	8.1(12)	41.6(62)	36.98(55)	13.4(20)
Fats (gm)	30	0(0)	2.7(4)	9.4(14)	13.4(20)	74.5(111)
Iron (mg)	20	16.8(25)	70.5(105)	8.7(13)	3.4(5)	0.7(1)
Calcium mg)	400	0.7(1)	0.7(1)	0.7(1)	14.8(22)	83.2(124)
Fibre (gm)	28	68.5(102)	31.5(47)	0(0)	0(0)	0(0)
β-carotene (µg)	3000	0.7(1)	20.1(30)	40.9(61)	26.8(40)	11.4(17)
Vit. C (mg)	40	4(6)	2.7(4)	3.4(5)	3.4(5)	86.6(129)

(b) Male

Nutrients	*RDA**	*%RDA*				
		< 25	*26-50*	*51-75*	*76-100*	*>100*
Energy (K.cal)	1750	0	15.68(16)	16.66(17)	57.84(59)	9.80(10)
Protein (gm)	60	0.98(1)	17.64(18)	53.92(55)	24.49(26)	1.96(2)
Fats (gm)	30	0	3.92(4)	9.80(10)	13.72(14)	72.54(74)
Iron (mg)	30	28.43(29)	62.74(64)	6.86(7)	1.96(2)	0
Calcium (mg)	400	0	0	1.96(2)	16.66(17)	81.37(83)
Fibre (gm)	20	70.58(72)	28.43(29)	0.98(10)	0	0
β-carotene (μg)	2400	0	9.80(10)	26.47(27)	31.37(32)	32.35(33)
Vit. C (mg)	40	2.94(3)	3.92(4)	0.98(1)	1.96(2)	90.19(92)

Source: Natarajan, 1991.

It was observed that type and location of the institutions did not show any difference in nutrient intake of elderly.

Data on males showed that more that 15 per cent subjects were able to meet >50 per cent of RDA for energy, protein and vitamin C. In case of fiber and iron, around 90 per cent subjects could meet only 50 per cent of RDA.

In all elderly subjects there was poor consumption of fruits and vegetables leading to very low intake of iron and fiber.

In the same study data on major health problems was collected through administration of checklist. Analysis of the data showed significant increase in the problems of oral cavity.

Table XII: Percentage of the female elderly subjects having major health problems

Health problems	*Age groups*			*Total*	*Chi-square Value*
	60-70 years (n=39)	*70-80 years (n=72)*	*>80 years (n=38)*	*(N=149)*	
Oral cavity	71.8(28)	84.7(61)	97.4(37)	84.6(126)	9.64**
GIT	35.9(14)	41.7(30)	55.3(21)	43.6(65)	3.15^{NS}
Respiratory	35.9(14)	41.7(30)	47.4(18)	41.6(62)	1.04^{NS}
Hepatobiliary	5.1(2)	1.4(1)	2.6(1)	2.7(4)	1.35^{NS}
Pancreas	0(0)	0(0)	5.3(5)	1.3(2)	5.92^{NS}
Cardiovascular	43.6(17)	59.7(43)	47.4(18)	52.3(78)	3.14^{NS}
Endocrine	17.9(7)	22.2(16)	23.7(9)	21.5(32)	0.42^{NS}
Genitourinary	48.7(19)	40.3(29)	47.4(18)	44.3(66)	0.92^{NS}
Locomotor problems	71.8(28)	72.2(52)	81.6(31)	74.5(111)	1.34^{NS}
Central nervous system	48.7(19)	48.6(35)	60.5(23)	51.7(77)	1.59^{NS}
Problems of reproductive organs	23.1(9)	29.2(21)	18.4(7)	24.8(37)	1.62^{NS}

In female elderly with age advancement, in more than half of the female population under study showed higher prevalence of locomotor problems, cardiovascular problem and problems of central nervous system as compared to other health problems. Similar findings were also noted by Mehta and Patel (2003) on local institutionalised elderly.

Following figure shows the prevalence of major illnesses among males.

Fig. I: Percentage of institutionalised male elderly showing major health problems

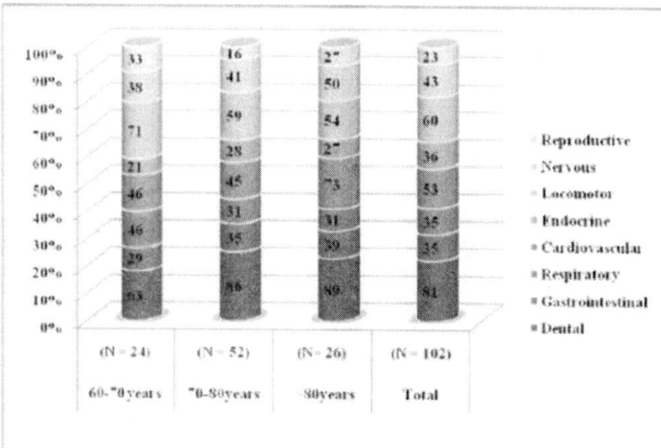

As can be seen from the above figure, dental problems were most prevalent in both the age group, followed by locomotor and cardiovascular problems.

Data on the minor illnesses of the institutionalised female elderly subjects living in old age homes of Gujarat is presented here.

Table XIII: Percentage of institutionalised female elderly having minor health problems (N=149)

Sr. no.	*Minor health problem*	*N*	*%*
1	Malaria	3	2
2	Infection-throat	8	5.4
3	Infection-skin	6	4
4	Infection-eyes	17	11.4
5	Vomiting	4	2.7
6	Diarrhea	5	3.4
7	Constipation	60	40.3
8	Acidity	51	34.2
9	Indigestion	14	9.4
10	Gas	54	36.2
11	Chest pain	22	14.8
12	No interest	12	8.1
13	Psychosomatic problem	2	1.3
14	Ulcers	11	7.4
15	Back pain	100	67.1

contd...

Sr. no.	*Minor health problem*	*N*	*%*
16	Headache	46	30.9
17	Muscle pain	22	14.8
18	Pain in joints	62	41.6
19	Dizziness	31	20.8
20	Dry skin	56	37.6
21	Trembling of limbs	32	21.5
22	Sleep disturbance	60	40.3
23	B.P fluctuation	15	10.1
24	Low mood	8	5.4
25	Lethargy	16	10.7
26	Appetite	53	35.6
27	Mood fluctuation	3	2
28	Pneumonia	0	0
29	Itching	40	26.8

Out of 149 female elderly, 85 per cent showed impaired vision, 70 per cent suffered from problems related to bones and memory loss whereas sleep disturbance was faced by 54 per cent of elderly females. Almost 40 per cent elderly women also had problems of bowel movements, dental problems and hearing problems.

Mental Profile

With increase in age, the elderly become more susceptible to physical disabilities and mental capabilities. Factors such as cultural pattern level of socio economic status, environment and social attitudes of the community play a vital role in mental well-being of the aged. There is change in their personal and social life. They are unable to pursue their occupation, lose their productivity and earning capacity. Feeling of being neglected by the children and loss of spouse may aggravate their depression status. Studies showed that 70 per cent of the mental morbidity is due to depression (Mehta and Shah, 2010).

In Gujarat old age homes out of 149 females, nearly one third of the population showed normal mental health as measured by MMSE scores. Though mental health was not affected age wise, the differences did exist in the mental health profile of inmates between the cities showing impact of environmental factors.

Cognitive impairment examination (CIT) showed fifty per cent of elderly female showed cognitive impairment which also varied with location.

With respect to males according to the parameters used for assessing the mental health, 62.7 per cent, 45.1 per cent, and 57.8 per cent of the subjects were in the normal category according to the GDI, MMSE and CIT scores respectively. No significant difference was observed between the different age groups and the four cities (Chauhan and Nair, 2010).

Recommendations

While analysing the overall scenario of the institutions and health profile of their inmates, the authors suggest following recommendations:

- Infrastructure facilities like dining facilities, recreation facility, bathroom, toilet and upholstery can be improved.
- Lift, telephone and banking facilities should be available all 24 hours.
- Facilities of transport, attendants for special needs and call for help during emergencies should be made available in all institutions.
- Inclusion of green leafy vegetables and fruits in the diet supplied by the institution should be made compulsory.
- Sick elderly and elderly with chewing or swallowing problems may be given diets considering their specific needs.
- Donors need to be educated so that institution kitchens are not loaded with sweets and fried foods. Instead donations of fruits, healthy food item or useful items may be encouraged.
- Physical and mental exercise may be promoted through professional worker employed only for this purpose by this institution.

- Joyful environment of activity like religion discussions, public lectures, film shows, entertainment programmes, music, etc. can be provided to enthuse elderly.
- Physical aids like spectacles, walker, stick, wheelchair, etc; should be available in the store wherever required.

Can institutionalised elderly themselves help in improving the health scenario?

Answer is "Yes", to some extent, it may be possible. Availability of resources cannot be controllable factor. However, if best can be used out of what is available, improvement can certainly occur. Knowledge regarding healthy practices in old age can be transmitted to every elderly. Since the food habits are deeply rooted, it is difficult to expect elderly to follow advice of family members or sometimes even care providers. However, if the advice comes from their own friend circles and if clear results are shown by following the health advice, it may be possible to convince the elderly to change his habits,

In this connection, our studies on elderly from local institution at Baroda, 2010 conducted showed interesting results. Positive change in the knowledge and practices of the institutionalised elderly was observed by imparting Nutrition Health Education to small group of female elderly which in turn percolated in the large group of other elderly inmates who were their co residents. Thus, elderly seem to be good change agents for imparting simple messages regarding health and nutrition of the elderly for their own peer group living around them.

There is ample scope for improvement in the facilities and infrastructure of old age homes currently present in major cities. Additional efforts are necessary to improve the nutritional status of the elderly inmates by bringing about behavioural changes and make provision for healthy diets, good recreation and health care.

Thus, while reviewing the issues discussed in this chapter, it can be suggested that:

1. Since the need for old age homes is increasing, both government and non government organizations should join hands together to run the old age homes.
2. Capacity building programs should be undertaken periodically to train the staff of old age homes and also the inmates.
3. Old inmates should be provided counseling facilities to cope up with social and psychological pressures.
4. Diet counseling centre, physiotherapy centre and recreation club should be a part of the infrastructure.

References

Bagchi K. (1999). Nutrition and ageing; an overview. In: Diet and Ageing: Exploring some facets. Kalyan Bagchi and Seema Puri (Ed), Society for Gerontological Research and Help Age India New Delhi: 7-18.

Chauhan K and Mehta P (2007), Health promotion for the aged through intervention with suitable foods and nutrient supplementation, M.Sc. Dissertation (unpublished), Dept. of Foods and Nutrition, The M.S.University, Baroda, India.

Chauhan K and Nair P (2010), Studies on nutrition and health profile of male elderly in old age homes in four major cities of Gujarat: Nutrition Health Education (NHE) intervention to female elderly as a change agents. M.Sc. Dissertation (unpublished), Dept. of Foods and Nutrition, The M.S. University, Baroda, India

Gurmeet Kaur (2010), Living pattern of individuals living in old age homes, Journal of Research and Development, Help Age India Publication, Delhi, Vol. 39, (2): 780-87.

Gurjeet Virk Sidhu (2010), Institutionalised older persons: A comparative study of old age homes. Help Age India, Journal of Research and Development, Vol. 16, (2): 24-31.

Goel S and Gupta M (2008), Quality of life of Elderly in Old Age homes in India: Impact of Interventions, Help Age India, Journal of Research and Development, Vol. 14, (3): 19-23.

Jamuna D (1998) Challenges of changing socioeconomic and psychological status of the aged. Help Age India: Research and Development Journal, Vol. 5 (1), 513.

Mehta P (1999).Diet, nutrition and health profile of elderly population of urban Baroda city, CF chapter: Book on Diet and Ageing edited by Dr. Kalyan Bagchi and Seema Puri , Society for Gerontological Research and Help Age India New Delhi: 63-71.

Mehta P and Limaye A (1999), A study on diet, nutrition and health profile of institutionalised and non-institutionalised elder lies of Baroda city (60 + years) M.Sc. Dissertation (unpublished), Dept. of Foods and Nutrition, The M.S. University, Baroda, India.

Mehta P and Patel N (2003), Effect of soy foods on health & nutritional status institutionalised elderly (unpublished) M.Sc. Dissertation, Dept. of Foods and Nutrition, Faculty of Home Science, The M.S. University of Baroda, India.

Mehta P and Shah H (2010), Studies on nutrition and health profile of female elderly in old age homes in four major cities of Gujarat: Nutrition Health Education (NHE) intervention to female elderly as a change agents. Unpublished master dissertation.

Mehta P, Patel K and Chauhan K (2009), Assessment of diet, nutrition and disease profile of elderly females residing in rural setting of Vadodara. Helpage India publication, Delhi, Vol. 17, (1): 5-14.

Mehta P, Chauhan K, Gandhi H, Shah K and Telang P (2010), Health promotion through nutritionally improved recipes for feeding vulnerable groups. Report submitted to Gujarat State Forest Development Corporation Limited, Vadodara, July 2010.

3

Stepping the Ladder of Ageing

I hope to die young, as late as possible

–Prof Sir Richard Dol

Healthy or successful ageing is the ideal situation in which people survive to an advanced age with their vigour and functional indępendence maintained and morbidity and disability compressed into a relatively short period after death (Campaign, 1998).

Centenarians are best model for studying healthy ageing and longevity as they already delay or escape diseases that would otherwise be lethal at younger ages (Event et al., 2003). According to Okinowacentarian study (1976–2003) with 560 centarians and elders (770 yrs), centarians in particular have experienced slower age related decline whereas it was found in contrast with the younger Okinawa's who lead a less healthy lifestyle and experienced higher mortality rates.

A fundamental challenge is to understand how centarians live longer and what specific biological, psychological and sociological characteristic they possess that would allow them to survive longer.

Studies on mortality profile of elderly show that proportion of people with chronic diseases raises decade by decade after 60 yrs (Prakash LJ, 1997). Prevalence of oral cavity was highest, followed by GIT, neurological, CVD and respiratory problems. Elderly are predisposed to malnutrition at later age because of loss of teeth and ill fitting or no denture. Moderate to severe anemia in older elderly is also a common finding (Mehta et al., 1997). Cataract, bronchitis, hypertension, constipation and arthritis are reported to be very common among elderly. Other problems which appear common after 7th decade are impaired vision, impaired hearing, locomotor problems frequent osteoporotic fractures, oral dryness, reduced salivary flow rate and flatulence.

Doty et al. (1984) tested smell identification ability in subjects ranging from 5 to 99 yrs of age and found that more than 60 per cent of subjects aged 65–80 yrs had major olfactory deficits and above the age of 80, this increased to more than 80 per cent.

There are many factors which contribute to healthy life in old age. Some of them are discussed below :

(a) Diet and Nutrition

Healthy diet plays a very important role in promoting and maintaining health of the elderly. Good nutrition helps in preventing or delaying the onset of age related illnesses. A good diet in later years helps both in reducing the risk of these diseases and in managing the diseases signs and symptoms which contributes to a higher quality of life enabling older people maintain their independence in activity. (Newman et al., 2006).

A study by Morris et al. (1996) on 3,718 subjects aged 65 years and above showed that high vegetables consumption can be associated with slower rate of cognitive decline with old age. Evans et al. (2008) carried out a study on 2889 subjects aged 65–102 yrs showed that vitamin E intake is associated with less cognitive decline with age. In a study on 100 elderly aged 50 - 70 yrs, it was found that 90 per cent depressed elderly had lowered the consumption of vitamin E, Vitamin B6 and vitamin B12 by 25 per cent of RDA (Mehta & laddu, 2002). Most of the studies conducted by our geriatric research team have reported much lower intake of food and nutrients as compared to RDA.

In earlier studies by Fischenetil (1995) and Willint et al. (1992), centenarians consume 20–30 per cent more caretenoids from food and consumed breakfast regularly than 60–80 year old elderly. Ortega et al. (2003) carried out a study on 168 elderly aged 65-90 years which revealed that subjects with satisfactory intellectual functions generally had a better diet in terms of adequate consumption of fatty acids, cholesterol and greater intake of vitamins. Mointosh et al. (1990) studied 424 non institutionalised individuals of both sexes, aged 50–100 yrs and revealed that 67 per cent of the subjects used nutritional supplements.

(b) Physical activity

Physical activity contributes to healthy living to a greater extent. In Russia labour is believed to be a major course of longevity (Dewan, 1994). The World Health Organisation (2004) has advocated for the promotion of participating in regular moderate intensity, physical activity from youth into old age.

Physical activity is protective for many ageing disorders and problems that affect the morbidity and mortality of elderly populations.

Bone health status of 60 elderly males with respect to 1000 mg calcium and 500 IU vitamin D_3 supplementation was studied for a period of 3 months showed a significant ($p \leq 0.05$) improvements in the BMD levels among group A and group B (30 subjects each). High significant ($p \leq 0.001$) improvement in the BMD levels of the subjects belonging to group A was observed, which received additional weight bearing exercise intervention besides the regular calcium and vitamin D_3 intervention (Chauhan and Pawar, 2013). Similar findings were noted among elderly female also with same type of intervention by Chauhan and Mistry, 2012.

Tanaka et al. (2000) conducted a study on 151 healthy men aged 18–77 yrs which showed that regular aerobic exercise lowers the risk of CVD. Kim et al. (2003) carried a study on 748 people aged 65 yrs and above which indicated high walking speed in daily life is a significant predictor of prolonged active life expectancy. Earlier study by Hakim et al. (1999) on 2678 subjects aged 71–93 yrs indicated that increase in distance walked reduces the incidence at CVD.

Ryan et al. (1994) carried out study on nearly one hundred elderly men and women and showed that high intensity resistance exercises is a feasible and effective means of counteracting muscle weakness and physical fragility in very old elderly. Another study by Blumenthan et al. (1991) on 101 elderly >60 yrs showed that exercise training may produce greater improvement in elderly with physical or emotional impairments.

A study on 932 men and 1067 females aged 50–89 yrs showed that exercises have less depressed mood (Silversteain et al., 2001).

Thus, physical activity is important protective factor for physical and mental health.

(c) Psychosocial Health

Old age is associated by a number of psychological, physiological and mental changes. Depression is more common with poor psychological well-being of older individual and is linked to their economic well-being, structural strains and constraints like low socio economic status and poor health and longevity.

A study reported by Buono et al. (1998) reported that positive attitude was responsible for longevity of individuals who live longer. The study included comparison of 38 centenarians for their psychophysical well-being with those of between 75–85 years and 88–99 yrs. The results revealed that centenarians complained less spontaneously about their health but declared having greater functional disability. The cognitive functions appeared to be reasonably well preserved and they had lower scores for anxiety and depression than their younger elderly counterparts. Older elderly reported greater satisfaction with life and with social and family relations than younger and elderly. Thus, the centenarians seemed to maintain a more positive attitude than their younger counterparts.

Stevens et al. (1999) found higher scores for memory in adults and elderly who were socially and physically more active than their counterparts. The breaking down of joint family system has taken away the social and economic security of the elderly and affective young social networks contributing to feeling of loneliness and bankruptcy in the elderly. It has been shown that loneliness, social and physical health are directly related to dietary adequacy and well-being of elderly (Walker et al. 1991)

Tijhuls (1999) reported that increased loneliness experienced by very old men was influenced by loss of a partner, moving into old age home or not feeling healthy.

Benneti (2002) reported that low levels of social engagement either have a direct effect on mortality or represent hidden health outcomes.

(d) Other factors

Cigarette smoking has a direct effect on body fat distribution as shown by the study on 765 men aged 43-85 yrs (Trois et al., 1991). A study by Ott et al. (2004) on 17,610 elderly showed that smoking accelerates cognitive decline in non dementia elderly. Earlier studies have also showed cigarette smoking and heavy drinking as major risk factors of diseases in elderly (Goldberg et al., 1980, Thin et al., 1997).

Religiousness has been found to have negative associations with rates of depression suicide and cognitive dysfunction (Ness et al, 2002). A study by Hill et al, (2005) on elderly showed that weekly church attendance may reduce the risk of mortality among older Mexican Americans.

A study on 3851 elderly by Helm et al (2000) indicated that older adults who participated in private religious activities before the onset of ADL impairment appear to have a survival advantage over those who do not.

It is believed that by exercising or doing yoga, one tends to appear younger by age and heart. Meditation is a powerful spiritual practice and regular act of meditation can help a great deal in one's spirituality developments (Thomsitt 2006, Shappire 2007).

It appears from the findings of studies reported in the literature that stress relieving practices like meditation and prayers combined with positive attitudes can result in good mental health in elderly leading to good longevity and better quality of life in old age.

In the light of current literature author's research team had undertaken studies on very old elderly to explore the situation under which they lived and secrets of their longevity. This was achieved by assessing the demography, nutritional status, dietary pattern, life style factors disease profile and health of 140 elderly belonging to various age groups of elderly (65 to 104 yrs).

The study also included comparison of the healthy elderly with the younger counterparts with health problems at an early age to look into the factors responsible for healthy ageing and longevity. Out of total of 140 elderly subjects, they were divided into two groups i.e. group A signifying elderly with poor fitness (65–84 yrs) and group B (i.e. elderly with good fitness (85 yrs) with 15 subjects in each group.

Data showed that majority of male elderly (88 per cent) were married, lived with their spouse's and majority received external help for daily activities from their spouse. On the other hand majority of female elderly were widows (58.4 per cent), lived with their families and a high percentage of them received external help from family members (67.6 per cent).

With regard to life style factors mean time spent for activity of daily living increased with advancement of age. Percentage of addicted subjects towards cigarette and bidi was also more in age groups of 65–74 yrs and 75–84 yrs as compared to their older counterparts. Majority of elderly males and females belonging to different age groups had moderate degree of anemia. Equal number (50 per cent) of total subjects had normal and abnormal glucose levels with highest prevalence (63.3 per cent) of normal levels in 93–104 yrs age group.

Table I: Mean time spent on different activities by subjects belonging to different age groups and both gender (mean ± s.d.)

Sr. No.	Activities	Age Groups (years)			
		65-74	75-84	86-92	93-104
1	**DAILY ACTIVITIES** (min.)				
	MALES	40.7± 2.26	43.8±1.95	45.6±1.76	48.6±1.55
	FEMALES	25.5±1.3	28.8±1.22	33.4±1.52	35±2.1
2	**LEISURE TIME** (min.)				
	MALES	122±1.59	128.2±1.65	130±1.54	135±1.34
	FEMALES	132.1±1.8	137±1.91	139.4±.77	142±1.52
3	**EXERCISE** (min.)				
	MALES	20±0.61	27.7±0.41	30.9±0.34	37.3±1.3
	FEMALES	20±2.1	23.2±2.9	15±1.8	18.7±1.19
4	**RELIGIOUS** (min.)				
	ACTIVITIES				
	MALES	22.6±1.6	20.8±1.32	35±1.1	27.9±0.9
	FEMALES	25.3±.7	20±1.2	33.9±0.88	35±0.74
5	**YOGA and MEDITATION (min.)**				
	MALES	5.2+1.5	6.8+1.76	18.7+1.5	14.3+1.82
	FEMALES	2.4+2.8	4.9+2.2	15.4+1.65	12.6+1.13

With respect to dietary intake, a significant difference was found between the nutrient intake of β - carotene, Folic acid and Vitamin C when compared to RDA between various groups. Data on food frequency and general dietary in formation showed that frequency of consumption of antioxidant rich food was irregular in age group of 65–74 yrs and 75–84 yrs. Majority of subjects (75 per cent) were vegetarians.

General health profile of the subjects revealed that majority of elderly in age groups of 75–84 yrs (62.5 per cent), 85–92 yrs (53.3 per cent) and 93-104 yrs (63 per cent) wore dentures. Fifty five per cent of subjects in 63–74 yrs age group and 75–84 yrs age group had pain in bones and 53.3 per cent elderly in 93–104 yrs age group experienced difficulty in standing.

Prevalence depression (as measured by GDI) was found to be higher in 75–84 yrs category cognitive impairment (as assessed by CIT) was found abnormal in 43.3 per cent of subjects in 93–104 yrs age group.

With respect to disease profile, the data showed that dental problems ranked first in 65–74 yrs where as bone related problem were highest reported in age group of 93+ yrs age group. In younger elderly, lethargy body aches and pain in joints were commonly reported whereas in older elderly aged 93+ yrs lack of appetite was the major complaint.

As mentioned earlier, an attempt was made to explore determinants at healthy ageing and longevity by comparing the elderly with poor fitness (group A) with the elderly with good fitness (group B). A significant difference between times spent for activities of daily living between the two groups for various activities were found.

Data on dietary intake showed that the consumption of Calcium, Vitamin C, Folic acid and Beta Carotene in elderly with poor fitness (group A) was significantly different (when compared with RDA) from elderly with good fitness (group B0 who had nutrient intake closer to RDA. Also subjects with good fitness (group B) had a more regular pattern of meal consumption than unfit elderly.

Thus, antioxidants rich but low calorie diet, regularity in meal consumption, moderate level of physical activity and involvement in activities like meditation and yoga were some of the determinants of achieving good health in later old age. Following points summarise the salient secrets which help in climbing the ladder of ageing.

- Consumption of antioxidants and calcium in required amount by elderly leading to their low morbidity profile and showing physical and mental fitness.
- Regular consumption of various meals maintains good nutrient status leading to positive effects of physical and mental well-being of the elderly. Active participation in various daily living activities by the elderly helps in keeping them fit and alert.
- Yoga, Meditation and religious activities help elderly to remain spiritually and physically healthy.
- Socialization and activities requiring mental efforts are a must.

Elderly who has been successfully climbing the ladder of ageing is truly living stress free life full of health, joy and eternal satisfaction.

References

Benetti K M (2002), Low levels of social engagement as a precursor of mortality among people in later life, Age and ageing, 31: 165-168.

Blumenthal JA, Emergy CF, Madden DJ, Schniebolk S, George LK (1991) Long term effects of exercise on psychological functioning in older men and women, Jr. of Gerontology, 46:6: 352-61.

Buono MD (1998) Quality of life and longevity. a study of centenarians Jr. Per. Soc Psy, 4: 388-390.

Campaign, 1998.

Chauhan and Mistry, (2012), A study on lifestyle factors, dietary profile and morbidity of elderly population of urban Vadodada in realtion to bone disorder: Calcium and vitamin D supplementation as a change agent on bone mineral density of elderly women. Vadodara: Department of foods and nutrition,

Faculty of family and community sciences. M S University Baroda, Vadodara.

Chauhan and Pawar, (2013), Assessment of bone health status and its risk factors of elderly male population of urban vadodara: Calcium and Vitamin D3 supplementation as a change agent on bone mineral density (BMD) of elderly men. Vadodara: Department of foods and nutrition, Faculty of family and community sciences.

Dewan and Freser M, (1994), Strong bones in later life: luxury or necessity? Bulletin of the world health organisation, 77 (5) : 416-122.

Doty RL, Golbe LI, McKeown DA (1984), Olfactory testing differentiates between progressive supranuclear palsy and idiopathic Parkinson's disease, Neurology 43:962-965.

Evans WJ et al. (2008), Exercise and nutrition needs of elderly people: effects on muscle and bone Gerodontology, 15: 1: 15-24

Event J, Lawler E, Bogan H and Perls T (2003) Morbidity profiles of centenarians: survivors, delayers and Escapers, Jr. of Gerontology, 58A (3): 232-237.

Fischen, Flint DM, Wahlqvist ML, Parikh AE (1995), The nutritional assessment of community and institutionalized elderly in Australia. Foods Nut. Notes Rev: 36:173-6.

Goldberg et al., Godfrey N, Kaiache A, (1980), Health needs of elder adults displaced to Sudan by warand famine: Questioning current targeting practices in health relief. Social science and medicine 28:707-713, CF: Symposium on nutrition and ageing in the developing world., Jr. of Nut. 131:24295-328.

Hakim A, Petrovitch H, Robert D, Lon R (1999) Effects of walking on mortality among non smoking elderly men, New England Jr. of Medicine, 338: 94-99.

Helm , Heller D et al (2000), Neurological disorder- Depression, Jr. Harvard Medical Association Nidus Publication, New York: 326-328.

Hill D, Ellison G, Ronald J (2005) Religious attendance and mortality: An 8 yrs follow up of older Mexican American, Jr. of Gerontology 60:S102-S109.

Kim et al, 2003.

Mehta P and Laddu K (2002), A study on diet, nutritional status and disease profile of elderly suffering from depression, Indian Jr. of Gerontology: 18: 250-257.

Mehta P, Sheth M, Vyas M (1997), Socio-demographic, Nutrition and Health profile of Indian elderlies (50-70 years) living in urban Baroda, India, Department monograph "Reaching the unreached", Department of Foods and Nutrition, The M.S. University of Baroda, Vadodara, India.

Mointosh et al., Meccoci P, Polidori MC, Troiano L, Cherubini A, Senin U (1990), Vegetarian nutrition, physical activity and athletic performance University of Brussels, Perugia, Italy.

Morris Clare, Evans Denis A, Tangeny Christine C, Julia L, Aggarwal T, Scherr A (1996) Relation of the tocopherol forms to incident Alzheimer disease and cognitive change, Dept. of Preventive Medicine.

Ness et al., 2002.

Newman. S and Tompkins. C (2006), A Case study reflecting Healthy Ageing in the U.S. Indian Journal of Gerontology, Vol. 20, No. 1 & 2, pp. 99-110.

Ortega M, Requejo M, Navia B (2003), Cognitive function in elderly people is influenced by Vitamin E status, Jr. Nut. 132:2065-2068.

Ott A, Anderson K, Lobo, Hofman A, Brayne C (2004), Effect of smoking on global cognitive function in non demented elderly, dept. of medical microbiology and infectious diseases, Netherlands.

Prakash L J (1997), Women and Ageing, Ind. Jr. Med Res., 106:369-408.

Ryan et al, 1994, Ryan and Shea (1996), Recognising depression in older adultsJr. Am Diet Asso. 96: 1-5.

Stevens F C J, Charles D Kaplan (1999), How ageing and social factors affect memory, Age Ageing 4 (28): 379-384.

Silverstein DK, Connor EB, Corbeau C (2001), Cross sectional and prospective study of exercise and depressive mood in the elderly, Am. Jr. of Clinical Nutrition, 153:6: 596-603.

Tanaka H, Dienno Frank A, Kevin D (2000), Ageing, habitual exercise and dynamic arterial compliance, Dept of kinesiology and Applied Physiology, University of Colorado at Boulder.

Thin et al., 1997.

Thomsitt, Thomas TP, Neal RR, Olshansky J, (2006), To Discover the Secrets of a Long Healthy and Happy Life, Journal of the American Medical Association,294:16:2086-2090.

TijhuisAR ,Jong DE, Fesken JM (1999), Changes in and factors related to loneliness in older men, The Zutpen Elderly Study, Age and Ageing, 28:491-495.

Troisi RJ, Heinold JW, Vokonas PS (1991), Cigarette smoking, dietary intake and physical activity: effects on body fat distribution- normative ageing study, American Journal of Clinical Nutrition, 53: 1104-1111.

Walker A (1991), The relationship between the family and the state in the care of older people Canadian Jr. on Ageing, 10:2: 94-112.

Willint and Willigen et al, (1992), The life scale: the development of a measure of successful ageing, In. Jr. Ger., 9:3: 83-90.

4

Mental Health and Ageing

> You are as young as your faith, as old as your doubt,
> as young as your self confidence, as old as your fear,
> as young as your hope, as old as your despair/
>
> **—Mac Arthur**

Ageing is a dynamic process that represents the molecular, biochemical, physiological and structural changes that take place in an individual following cessation of growth.

Continuous efforts since 1960s are being carried on in the field of geriatrics. Several theories had been postulated. First one is the wear and tear theory explaining that wear and tear takes place owing to free radical activity and another theory describes ageing to be genetic i.e. programmed into the organism. Various integrated theories have come around in which free radical damage to DNA is seen to result in altered nervous system. A free radical is an atom or group of atoms possessing one or more unpaired electrons causing the normal ageing process.

Elderly individuals face a higher risk of developing mental as well as physical morbidity. While there is increasing concern about medical facilities, hardly any attention is paid at mental health issues. The vulnerability of elderly to mental problems is due to ageing of brain, physical problems, socio-economic factors, cerebral pathology, emotional attitude and family structure. Mental illnesses that predominantly affect older people include memory loss, depression, dementia and many others. There is estimation of 2.8 million adult with common and severe mental disorders at any given time in Gujarat. In light of these facts main focus of this chapter deals with information related to two major disorders i.e. depression and dementia. Results of some studies conducted by authors with the team of their department (Department of Foods and Nutrition, The M.S. University of Baroda, Vadodara, Gujarat) are also highlighted in this chapter.

Most recently, the field of Global Mental Health has emerged as the area of study, research and practice that places a priority of improving mental health. As per WHO report (2001), mental health problems are among the most important contributors to the global burden of disease and disability. At the global level, mental health problems currently are said to be 8 per cent of the global burden of diseases and more than 15 per cent of adult in the developing societies are estimated to suffer from mental illness. Desijarlais et al, 1995). Mental disorders are projected to increase to 15 per cent of the global disease burden by the year 2020 (Lewis and Areya, 2001).

In India, according to a north Indian survey, the rate of psychiatric morbidity is 82 per cent per 1000 population. Prabhu and Raghuram (1987), estimated more than 30 million individuals suffering from mental illness every year and that 0.175 million individuals are added every year.

Amongst all other groups, health needs of the growing number of older people pose a serious challenge as older individuals are frail, disabled or cognitively impaired. There are an estimated 4 million old people with serious mental disorders and another 25-30 million with minor disturbances. The prevalence of mental disorders is likely to rise as life expectancy increases (Vishwanathan and Wetzel, 1993). Depression and dementia are the most common disorders in old age illnesses. Therefore these two disorders have been covered here along with few other mental illnesses.

Depression

Depression poses a major public health challenge in the coming years. According to WHO estimates, within the next 20 years, recurrent depressive disorder will be the second most serious cause of morbidity in the world. Available literature indicates women and older people being more at risk of depression due to physiological and socio-cultural reasons (Joshi et al., 2005). The vulnerability of older women to depression is increased due to the process of ageing, poor health, under nutrition, decreasing ability to function, loss of spouse and other significant relations, feeling of isolation, insecurity, economic dependence, decreasing importance in the family and so forth. The problem of depression in older women may be more complex due to the difficulty in recognising depression in older persons and their double disadvantage of being elderly persons at the same time. There is therefore an urgent need for interventions to combat depression in older persons—women in particular. In view of this, it is important to understand the role that various psycho-social, health and nutrition related factors associated with depression play in the onset of depression.

In this regard, the findings of the project on "Mental health and ageing" undertaken by the investigators (including the authors) at the Maharaja Sayajirao University of Baroda, (2005) are worth mentioning. The project had a research as well as intervention component. Initial part of the study examined the prevalence of mental disorders as reported in the psychiatric disorders. The second section included in-depth study at psychological and cultural aspects of their lives as well as the health and nutrition status. An intervention study was also carried out on depressed elderly women with folic acid supplementation. Findings of this project are discussed briefly to understand the magnitude of the disease and its impact on health of elderly women in Gujarat.

Prevalence of Mental Disorders in Gujarat

Evidence from retrospective and prospective data. In all 17,710 records were obtained from public (4,775 records) and private hospitals and clinics (12,935, of which 10,908 were retrospective data, obtained from year 2000 to 2002) and 6,800 were prospective data. The data from six cities of Gujarat on clients of mental health sciences showed that:

- Depression and Schizophrenia are the most prevalent mental health disorders followed by anxiety disorders and bipolar disorders.
- Mental retardation and seizures are more in younger group whereas dementia is more prevalent in older age group.
- Depression is higher in women than in men. Mental health problems of women also seem to be under reported.

Depression in Adult and Older Women

Phase 2 of the project included study of prevalence of depression in adult and ageing women from free living population for which in-depth interviews were conducted with women over 40 yrs of age in vadodara city.

Vadodara city has divided into 25 areas which were further classified into locations representing different income groups. The subjects were screened on the basis of Beck's Depression Inventory (BDI) to obtain a sample of 180 women who were selected for in-depth interview.

Data on the psychosocial aspect of women showed that living arrangements are changing from joint to nuclear families. Feeling of loneliness and insecurity was present in women who were away from families or were widow. In this study, a very high percentage of older women have reported experience of abuse or neglect by husbands or daughter-in-law. Women were found to cope with neglect, abuse, loneliness or isolation by crying or tolerating.

In elderly, loss of appetite, fatigue and under nutrition along with other nutritional deficiencies have been found to be more prevalent. Weight loss is known to be associated with depression. Therefore, this study also investigated health and nutrition related aspects in depressed elderly women. It was observed that no depressed women had better water consumption compared to their non depressed counterparts. An exploratory study among women of Boston reported that depressed women had much lower water consumption as compared to non depressed women. (Benton and Cook, 1991). The most common reasons for limiting fluid intake was 'laziness', 'limited mobility', 'workload' and 'forgetfullness' in drinking water. Women who were elderly and had limited mobility had lower intake of water.

The study showed more regular meal pattern (Breakfast, lunch, snacks and dinner) in case of non depressed elderly subjects as compared to depressed elderly.

Skipping meals was common in depressed women, particularly breakfast. Older women reported reasons for skipping meals as lack of support from the family, quarrels, arguments and conflict in the family, lack of choices in matter of food cooked, physical disability or locomotor complaints, financial dependence on other family members and customarily practices on account of widowhood. Research that compared three studies involving breakfast, memory function and blood glucose levels concluded that eating breakfast benefited the memory. Reduction of food intake due to loss of appetite, low mood and other psychological reasons has been associated with depression. In this study, as shown in table 4.1 below reduction in food consumption due to lost appetite, low mood, development of aversion or dislike was higher in women in the age group of 40–60 yrs and above 60 yrs (80-87 per cent). For low income group women, besides loss of appetite and low mood, inability to afford food of their choice and no choice in their food pattern were main reasons for reduction in food consumption. The study also showed reduction in food consumption such as cereals, milk and milk products, fried foods, ghee, masalas, pickles, sweets and sugar.

Table I: Percentage of subjects showing reasons of reduction of food intake.

Reasons	*Depressed*						*Non-depressed*
	40-60 yrs			*>60 yrs*			*>60 yrs*
	LIG n=30	*MIG n=30*	*HIG n=30*	*LIG n=30*	*MIG n=30*	*HIG n=30*	*MIG n=20*
	%	%	%	%	%	%	%
Lost appetite	86.7	60.0	66.7	86.7	60.0	83.3	25.0
No mood	86.7	53.3	63.3	86.7	37.9	83.3	-
Developed aversion/ dislike	58.6	44.8	46.7	75.0	50.0	63.3	10.0
Any other	80.0	100	100	87.5	22.2	87.5	50.0

As measured by 24 hr dietary recall method, data collected was further divided into two different age groups for depressed subjects and attempt was made to compare the dietary intake with elderly non depressed subjects. The following table II shows the intake of various nutrients of subjects belonging to different income groups.

Table II: Nutrient intake of depressed and non-depressed elderly.

Nutrients	**Depressed**						**Non-depressed**
	40-60 yrs			**>60 yrs**			**>60 yrs**
	LIG n=30	**MIG n=30**	**HIG n=30**	**LIG n=30**	**MIG n=30**	**HIG n=30**	**MIG n=20**
Energy (Kcal)	1264 + 303	1832 + 369	1903 + 541	1012 + 357	1343 + 334	1305 + 337	1906 + 341
Protein (gms)	22 + 10	35 +10	35 + 10	19+ 8	30+9	27+8	56+9
Fat (gm)	18 + 7	28+ 8	29+ 11	18+ 8	23+ 8	28+ 8	45+ 9
Iron (mg)	19 + 6	28+ 9	22+ 9	14+ 9	17+ 7	20+ 8	38+ 6
Folic acid (ug)	83 + 37	102+32	80+39	59+29	53+17	70+37	141+23
Vitamin B6 (mg)	1.47 +1.16	1.76+1.05	1.50+0.69	0.90+0.91	0.96+0.70	1.18+0.53	2.98+0.90

Nutrients	Depressed						Non-depressed
	40-60 yrs			>60 yrs			>60 yrs
	LIG n=30	MIG n=30	HIG n=30	LIG n=30	MIG n=30	HIG n=30	MIG n=20
Calcium (mg)	189 + 111	266+94	235+76	177+86	228+93	255+86	508+76
Choline (mg)	23 + 10	24+12	28+11	20+8	18+9	27+9	46+11
Isoflavone (mg)	35+ 14	40+13	41+10	31+12	31+11	40+11	73+9
Tryptophan (mg)	120 +30	143+36	136+39	115+30	121+28	133+34	276+43
Methionine (mg)	373 +127	481+116	387+150	343+136	409+115	443+118	657+45
Phenylalanine (mg)	138 +54	148+44	130+44	110+37	125+36	113+34	249+26
Vitamin C (mg)	22 +13	29+10	25+8	23+8	17+8	23+8	55+8
Potassium (mg)	1720 +690	1826+882	1905+690	1990+690	1930+799	2016+1074	5219+855
Selenium (ug)	8.09+10.51	6.79+8.14	8.53+9.00	7.33+7.09	7.47+9.86	6.89+6.40	42.75+12.15

Data in table II depicted that older depressed women showed lower nutrient intake as compared to their younger counterpart across all income groups. This was more true for middle class older depressed women where significant difference in nutrient intake with respect to energy, iron, folic acid, tryptophan, methionine and vitamin C was observed ($p \leq 0.05$). Also, main key nutrients responsible for depression i.e. choline, seleneium and isoflavone intake was significantly lower among depressed older group as compared to their non depressed counterparts.

Studies conducted earlier by the author's team also showed association of low food intake with poor cognitive function (Mehta and Laddu, 2001, Mehta and Shah, 2006 and Mehta et al, 2010).

Thus, there are factors in a person's background that constitute a risk for depression and life events such as bereavements, acute physical illness of self or someone close, major financial crisis, negative interactions with family members or friends etc., other chronic stressors are declining health, dependence, socio economic decline, marital problems, problem at work, retirement or loneliness and isolation.

Mental health of women is also governed by factors such as cultural factors, experience of violence, neglect or abuse, power structure, stressful life events. In this connection, effect of power structure, loneliness and isolation, stress and isolation were studied by author's team on depressed subjects which are presented below. All the psychosocial factors mentioned here showed significant impact on nutrient intake of women with depression.

Table III: Power structure and calorie intake of depressed women (N=180)

Power structure	*Calorie intake Mean value*	*f- ratio*	*f- value*
Satisfied (n= 30)	1433± 501	0.6028	0.5484
Dissatisfied (n=100)	1393 ± 491		
Not sure (n=50)	1530 ± 470		

It can be seen from the above table that none of the categories of satisfaction with existing power structure showed significant difference with the calorie intake of depressed women though apparently women who were satisfied with the existing power structure within the family had better calorie intake.

Table IV: Isolation and calorie intake of women with depression (N=180)

Isolation	*Calorie intake Mean value*	*t- value*	*p- value*
Always + sometimes (n=130)	1077 + 107.5	4.41* 0.000	
Never (n=50)	1112 + 101.1		

*Significant at $p<0.05$

As can be seen from table IV, the association of isolation and calorie intake were significant ($p\leq0.05$) in depressed women, which means that women who ranked higher for isolation on the BDI also had lower calorie intake. From the study it can be mentioned that when women were being interviewed on the psychosocial aspects they were asked what they were doing when they felt isolated. Their response was loss of appetite, no mood to eat. This explains the low calorie intake by women who experienced feelings of isolation.

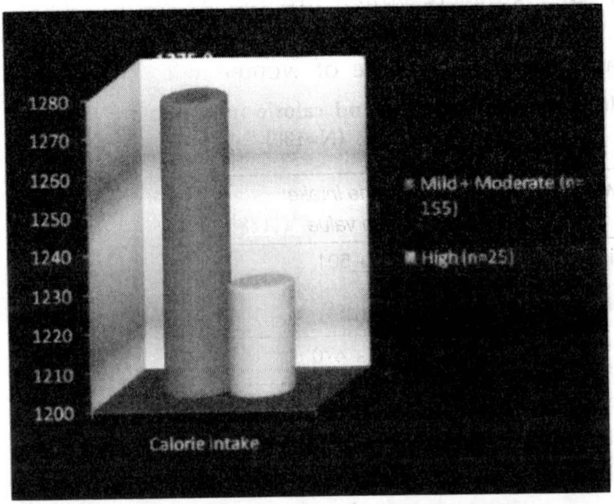

Fig. I: Level of stress and calorie intake of depressed women

Thus, issue of depression in elderly is a critical one and more so for elder women who feels prey to difficult social situations indicating the need for taking concrete steps for creating awareness amongst elderly and their caregivers regarding depression and its predisposing factors.

DEMENTIA

The mental disorders that are frequently encountered include dementia and mood disorders. Other disorders include neurotic and personality disorders, drug and alcohol abuse, delirium and mental psychosis.

As mentioned above, old age by default brings certain issues that these people need to deal with. Apart from the decline in physical stamina, ageing does reduce some cognitive ability in an individual. Few of the common cognition problems related to age are forgetfulness, inability to think quickly and difficulty in recalling past incidences. Decrease in cognitive ability is one of the major challenges that most of the elder people face. Cognition is the ability of an individual to think and act accordingly to the accepted norms. Cognition generally refers to the mental ability of an individual. Impairment in cognition in simple terms would be a delay or improper function of an individual's mental ability, which affects its thoughts, language and functioning. Mild cognitive impairment refers to the presence of cognitive impairment that is not severe enough to meet the criteria of dementia. Dementia is one of the most common critical problems related to ageing which ultimately results in one's death after complete memory loss. Prevalence of dementia which is characterised by a decline in memory, language and other cognitive functions is high in the older population and studies show that it is more prevalent in women than in men (Rashid, 2012).

According to the World Health Organisation, the South-East Asia Region (WHO SEAR), the dementia mortality rate for India is 13.5 per 100,000 males and 11.1 for 100,000 females. Global Burden of Disease report 2006, dementia is the third leading cause contributors to years if life lost due to disability (YLD) in the elderly in low-income and middle-income countries. The WHO Report estimated that dementia is the second highest source of disease burden after tropical diseases.

The prevalence of dementia among individuals aged 71 and older was 13.9 per cent, comprising about 3.4 million individuals in the USA in 2002. The corresponding values for AD were 9.7 per cent and 2.4 million individuals. Dementia prevalence increased with age, from 5.0 per cent of those aged 71–79 years to 37.4 per cent of those aged 90 and older. (US National Library of Medicine National Institutue of Health, 2007). Jotheeswaran et al. (2010) showed that prevalence of dementia was high in women as compared to men in India. Presently, an estimated 3.7 million Indian people aged over 60 have dementia (2.1 million women and

1.5 million men). The prevalence of dementia increases steadily with age and higher prevalence is seen among older women than men.

Mild Cognitive Impairment is a common psychiatric problem among the elderly. Various terms have been employed to characterise the cognitive decline associated with ageing, including benign senescent forgetfulness, age-associated memory impairment, and age-associated cognitive decline. (Heather and Anderson, 2012). Mild cognitive impairment (MCI) is an intermediate stage between the expected cognitive decline of normal ageing and the more serious decline of dementia. It can involve problems with memory, language, thinking and judgment that are greater than normal age-related changes (Mayo, 2012). Cognition declines with older age. Longitudinal studies report conversion rates of mild cognitive impairment to a diagnosis of dementia of approximately 10 per cent per year.

For elderly, mental health conditions are an important cause of morbidity and mortality. Thus, it is not surprising that with one in five individuals over age 65 are suffering from mental disorders, and the number of older adults with psychiatric disorder is expected to double in next 30 years. (Jeste *et al.*, 1999).

Dementia can be defined as a serious loss of cognitive ability in previously unimpaired person. It's an on-specific illness syndrome in which affected areas of cognition may be memory, attention, language and problem solving. Dementia can be categorised as:

1. **Senile Dementia:** This is a mental disorder that accompanies brain degeneration and occurs in old age.
2. **Pre-senile Dementia:** It's a disorder associated with the degeneration of brain earlier in life.

Memory functions that decrease when age increases include the following:

1. **Working Memory:** Holding and manipulating information in the mind, as when reorganising a short

list of words into alphabetical order verbal and visuospatial, working speed, memory, and learning, with visuospatial cognition more affected by ageing than verbal cognition.

2. **Episodic Memory:** Personal events and experiences.
3. **Processing Speed.**
4. **Prospective memory:** The ability to remember to perform an action in the future.
5. **Recollection.**

Some of the nutritional risk factors associated with ageing are lonely eating, inability to obtain right foods, changing food preferences due to degeneration of sensory capability, functional impairments and illness and also lack of awareness of changing age-related nutrition needs.

There are so many causes of mild cognitive impairment in elderly such as ageing of brain, genetic factors, nutritional deficiencies especially antioxidant vitamins, thiamine, folate, vitamin B_{12} and Omega-3 fatty acids, hormonal changes, alcoholism, obesity, drug abuse, Parkinson's disease, Huntington's disease, severe brain trauma, brain infections, unregulated diabetes mellitus or thyroid disorders. Thus it can be said that impaired cognition is never normal, loss of cognitive ability always represents serious disease that is at times irreversible and should always be promptly evaluated.

There are various ways used for treating mild cognitive impairment. Studies described before in the chapter showed that the deficiency of nutrients and development of MCI have a positive relation. The potential impact of dietary manipulation in the maintenance of physical and cognitive function between middle and old age has profound consequences for optimization of health, independence and well-being for later years. Thus nutrient intervention is thought to be one of the treatments to improve the cognitive function. And one of the main nutrients is vitamin B_{12} as it plays a very crucial role in brain development.

Vitamin B_{12} is found only in foods of animal origin like milk, meat, or eggs. Strict vegans who consume no animal-based foods need to supplement their diet with vitamin B_{12} to meet the body's need for this nutrient. Vitamin B_{12} is needed to maintain the outer coating, called the myelin sheath, on nerve cells. Inadequate myelin results in nerve damage and impaired brain function. Vitamin B_{12} deficiency can go undetected in individuals for years, but it eventually causes low blood iron, irreversible nerve damage, dementia, and brain atrophy.

There is long standing clinical evidence that Vitamin B_{12} deficiency causes neuronal dysfunction in the form of dementia, peripheral neuropathy, or sub acute combined degeneration. Vitamin B_{12} is crucial for the synthesis or utilization of important neuro-factors including monoamines, melatonin and serotonin. B_{12} is absolutely critical for the function and maintenance of nerves themselves. B_{12} is needed for methylation reactions that maintain these cells, and enable them to function. The high prevalence of likely metabolically significant vitamin B_{12} deficiency in the elderly is associated with lower cognitive function scores and particularly with lower scores of language comprehension and expression.

Trials suggest that Vitamin B_{12} deficiency is not the primary cause in most of demented people, but they do not exclude the possibility that Vitamin B_{12} deficiency contributes to dementia and its symptomatology. Therefore, in a study carried out on elderly women with Mild Cognitive Impairment (MCI) attempt was made by author for imparting intervention of Vitamin B_{12} injections (Thakker and Chauhan, 2012). Studies on ageing and mental health indicate a need for appropriate interventions.

In above referred study was carried out in two phases. In first phase 350 elderly men and women from free living population of Vadodara were screened for MCI using Mini Mental State Examination tool (MMSE, source Folestein, 1975) and Cognitive Impairment Test (CIT, source Katzman et al., 1983). Of which 250 subjects falling in the category of MCI (MMSE score between 21-26) were enrolled for the study. In phase II, 60 elderly women with MCI were purposively selected with age and scores matched. Thirty subjects were intervened with Vitamin B_{12} injection (1500 mcg once a week) and rest 30 subjects formed control group without intervention.

The findings of the formative research showed that MMSE and Age was slightly negatively correlated and was significant $p \leq 0.05$ levels. CIT and Age was slightly positively correlated but was not found significant. The frequency of consumption of milk and milk products was high in both the age groups (96.4 per cent) and low intakes of omega 3 rich foods and non-vegetarian foods in older age group as compared to younger elder age group. 76.8 per cent people suffered from memory loss in terms of recent events, past events, numbers, name and address of close friends. It was found that males were sociable and women were more reserved in both the age group. Mean age and screening scores are presented in table.

Table V: Mean MMSE, CIT scores and age of MCI subjects

Mental Health	*60-75 years*		*76-85 years*		*Total*
	Males (n=70)	*Females (n=151)*	*Males (n=15)*	*Females (n=14)*	*N=250*
MMSE	24.22± 1.64	23.71± 1.64	23.33±1.67	22.78±1.76	23.78±1.67
CIT	13.02±2.07	13.80±2.70	14.8±2.88	14.28±2.86	13.67±2.59
Age	67.01±4.33	68.88±4.02	80.33±3.55	80.14±2.24	67.26±6.23

Results of the intervention phase showed beneficial effect of Vitamin B_{12} as depicted in following tables and figure.

Table VI: Mean MMSE and CIT scores of subjects belonging to control and experimental group

Sr. no	*Mental health*	*Control group (n = 30)*		*t value*	*Experimental group (n = 30)*		*t value*
		Pre (A)	*Post (B)*		*Pre (C)*	*Post (D)*	
1.	**MMSE**	23.83 ±1.62	23.6 ±1.77	1.36(A+B) 0.33(A+C)	23.96 ±1.47	25.46 ±1.60	7.88***(C+D) 4.23***(B+D)
2.	**CIT**	13.7 ±2.24	13.63 ±1.92	0.46(A+B) 0.94(A+C)	13.2 ±1.60	9.8 ±1.77	8.5***(C+D) 8.04***(B+D)

As can be seen from the above table, there was a significant ($p \leq 0.001$) improvement among the experimental group where improvement in the scores of MMSE (significantly increased level) and CIT (significantly decreased level) were observed (paired t test). There was significant ($p \leq 0.001$) improvement also observed between the two group's post data (student t test). No change was observed in control group.

Hundred per cent subjects shifted from mild to normal level of vitamin B_{12} after intervention, whereas in control group no change was observed, where as 100 per cent subjects shifted from at risk to normal level of mean corpuscular volume after intervention with vitamin B_{12}, whereas no change was observed in control group.

Attempt was made to correlate intake of vitamin B_{12} with serum B_{12} levels and the result is presented in following table and graph.

Table VII: Correlation of vitamin B_{12} with serum B_{12} levels of the subjects

Sr. No.	*Indices*	*Mean (n=60)*
1	Serum vitamin B_{12}	153.8±43.02
2	Vitamin B_{12} intake	0.276±0.17
3	Pearson correlation	0.184

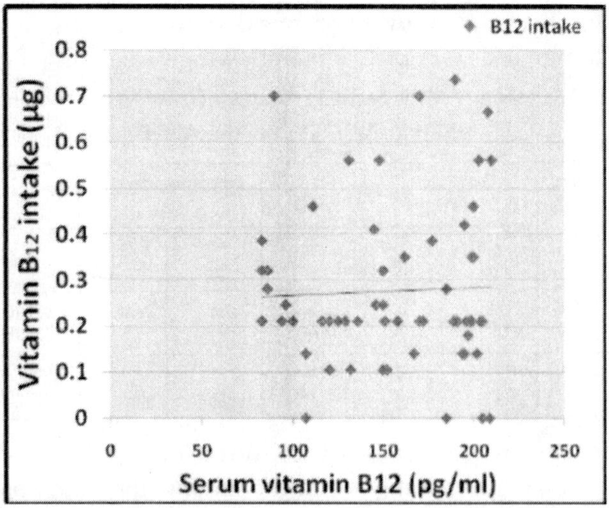

As revealed in the above scattered diagram weak positive correlation was observed between serum vitamin B_{12} and vitamin B_{12} intake. Following recommendations could be made from the study results.

- A need for proper treatment for age related disorders affecting mental health should also be emphasised
- To encourage vitamin B_{12} rich foods in the diet and for purely vegetarian people, a need to emphasise vitamin B_{12} supplementation for long period of time
- Regular check up of serum vitamin B_{12} in a definite period of time to avoid vitamin B_{12} deficiency after the age of 40 years
- To encourage mental health activity in elderly subjects which help to maintain healthy cognitive health
- A need to detect subjects for mild cognitive impairment after age of 50 years from free living population, early detection can avoid the deterioration of cognitive impairment.

Many other interventional strategies were also being studied for its beneficial impact on reducing the mental health problems amongst the elderly like use of herbs like ashwagandha, shankhpushpi, foods like soy, ragi and flaxseeds (Chauhan and Mehta, 2007, Mehta et al., 2010, Kansara and Chauhan, 2012).

References

1. Benton D., Cook R. 1991: The impact of selenium supplementation on mood. *Biol Psychiatry*; 29: 1092–1098.
2. Chauhan and Mehta, 2007: Health promotion for the aged through intervention with suitable foods and nutrient supplementation. PhD Dissertation (Unpublished), Department of Foods and Nutrition, The M.S.University, Baroda, India.
3. Dave P and Mehta P. 2008: Mental Health and Ageing: An important correlates, Kalpaz Publications, New Delhi.
4. Desjarlais, R., Eisenberg, L., Good, B. and Kleinman, A. 1995: World Mental Health: Problems and priorities in low-income countries. New York: Oxford University Press.
5. Folstein MF, Folstein SE and McHugh PR, 1975: Grading the cognitive state of patients for the clinician," J Psychiatry Res, 12(3): 189-98.
6. Heather, S and Anderson, 2012: Mild Cognitive Impairment, Medscape References, pp 1-8.
7. Jeste, D.V., Alexopoulous G.S., Bartels S.J., Cummings, J.L. et al., 1991. Consensus Statement on the Upcoming Crisis in Genatric Mental Health, Arch Gen. Psychiatry, 56 (9): 848-53.
8. Joshi K, Kumar R and Avasthi A. 2005: Morbidity profile and its relationship with disability and psychological distress among elderly people in Northern, India, Int J Epidemiol; 32 (6) 988-90.
9. Jotherswaran, A.J., Williams, J.D., and Prince M.J., 2010, The Predictive Validity of the Dementea diagnosis in Chennai: 3 year follow up study, Alzhermer Disease Association Disorder, 24 (3): 296-302.
10. Kansara, K and Chauhan, K, 2012: Effect of faxseeds on health and Nutritional status of institutionalised elderly of Vadodara, Unpublished master dissertation, Department of Foods and Nutrition, The M.S. University, Baroda, India.

11. Katz man R, Brown T, Field P et al., 1983: "Mini-Mental State: A Practical Method for grading the cognitive state of patients for the clinician," J Psychiatry Res, 12 (3): 189-98.
12. Lewis, G. and Araya, R. 2001: Classification, Disability and the Public Health Agenda. *British Medical Bulletin*, 57, 3-15.
13. Mayo, Q. 2012: Mild Cognitive Impairment, Mayo Foundation for Medical Education and Research.
14. Mehta P and Laddu K, 2002: A study on diet, nutritional status and disease profile of the elderly suffering from depression. In J Ger 16: 250-257.
15. Mehta P, Chauhan K and Purohit S, 2010: A study on nutrition and health of depressed adult and older men of Baroda city: Impact of herbal intervention (Brahmi) on depression in elderly men with impaired mental function, In J GerVol. 24, No. 1, pp. 49-58.
16. Mehta P and Shah A, 2006: A study on nutrition and health of depressed adult and older women of Baroda city: Impact of herbal intervention (Brahmi) on depression in elderly women with impaired mental function (Unpublished) M.Sc. Dissertation, M.S. University, Baroda.
17. Prabhu, G.G. and Raghuram,A, 1987: Mental Health in India in India. *Encyclopaedia of Social Work in India*, 2, 188-189 (published by Ministry of Welfare, New Delhi).
18. Rashid, A. K, 2012: Cognitive Impairment Among The Elderly Malays Living In Rural Malaysia, Med Jr Malaysia, pp. 186-89.
19. Thakker, R and Chauhan, K, 2012: Situational analysis of diet, nutrition and disease profile of elderly women with mild cognitive impairment: Impact of Vitamin B_{12}, Unpublished master dissertation, Department of Foods and Nutrition, The M.S.University, Baroda, India.
20. US National Library of Medicine National Institutue of Health, 2007: Prevalence of Dementia in the United States: The Ageing, Demographics, and Memory Study, Neuroepidemiology.
21. Vishwanathan, N., and Wetzel, Janice, W, 1993 in Mane, Purnima and Gandevia, katy, Y (eds) Mental Health in India: Issues and concerns. Bombay: Tata Institute of Social Sciences 43-69.
22. W.H.O. World health Report, 2001: Global burden of diseases, Geneva, Switzerland.

5

Guidelines for Diet and Nutritional Disorders in Elderly

> "Growing older is part of God's Plan". You can't "Hold back the dawn OR "Stop tides from flowing" OR "Keep a rose from withering" and Time cannot be halted in its swift - Endless fight for AGE.
>
> –**Unknown**

Ageing is an inevitable process. However, many issues of an ageing population can be overcome, delayed or prevented by correcting the life style factors. Diet and nutritional status play greater role than any other factors in determining the health of the aged individual.

It is being increasingly realised that diet plays a vital role in the ageing process. Certain types of foods can accelerate the ageing process during which diet related degenerative diseases are superposed with high mortality rate. On the other hand, there are specific foods and nutrients which can slow down the ageing process, prevent the onset of diet related chronic degenerative diseases thereby ensuring healthy ageing. However, certain diseases are caused purely due to nutrient deficiencies or over nutrition.

Some of the common nutritional disorders are osteoporosis, iron & folate deficiency anemia, obesity. Apart from these conditions, constipation and dental disorders are also very common conditions which require only dietary modifications. Diabetes, Cardiovascular diseases, hypertension and other medical conditions like cancer are not discussed in this chapter though these conditions are highly prevalent in elderly population. However, some tips for use in such conditions are also discussed here given in Appendix – (Tips on diets in such conditions).

Considerations for Normal Diet of Elderly

With biological ageing process, there are associated physiological changes in the body, changes in food preferences and food and nutrition intake.

With ageing process there are several changes which affect the diet of elderly. Reduced metabolism, loss of teeth, difficulty in mastication, alterations in taste buds, gastric dysfunctions and reduced intestinal mobility are such changes. There are several studies conducted in India assessing dietary intake and nutritional status of elderly living under different situations and most of the studies show that socio demographic attributes have great bearing on nutrition and health status of elderly. In this region of Gujarat. Baroda study reported by the authors in 1999 and subsequent research studies conducted so far by their team have indicated that socio demographic factors like income, living arrangement and certain lifestyle factors such as activity pattern and psychosocial aspects have profound influence on diet and nutrition profile of elderly subjects.

One striking feature in the outcome of all studies conducted by authors team since over two decades is that there appears a gross dietary inadequacy in terms of energy, calcium, iron, carotene and other important nutrients in free living elderly population as well as institutionalised elderly (Mehta et al., 2010 and Dhapola and Mehta, 2009). Elderly in religious order have shown encouraging diet pattern (Vasavda and Mehta 2003).

It is needless to point out that meal pattern and type of diet can not be ignored to protect health and well-being of the elderly.

There are some suggestions for the caregivers of elderly.

- Plenty of water/fluid needs to be included in the diet of elderly (more than 6 glasses).
- Three to four meals per day are appropriate. Fixed timings of meals may be maintained.
- Ensure adequate consumption of dairy products, protective foods like fruits and vegetables and cereals in the diet. Include whole grain cereals, sprouts and fiber rich foods in the diet.
- Avoid dry meals. Always add some beverage in the menu.
- Skipping of meals should be avoided.
- Special needs of elderly in disease conditions like hypertension and diabetes may be considered.
- Encourage the elderly members to eat with other members of the family.
- Include plenty of salads, soups and juicy fruits in the diet.
- Specific place for specific foods in the plate (like clock) may be maintained for serving very old elderly with poor eyesight.
- Avoid heavy meals and late night dinners.

As a general guideline adequate consumption of fruits and vegetables, whole grain, dairy products (non-fat) may be included in the diet of elderly where as "White poison" i.e. Ghee, Sugar, Salt, Oil can be controlled depending upon the physical condition.

For diabetic patients, apart from increased physical activity and maintenance of ideal body weight, carbohydrates such as sugar and starchy foods like potato and rice may be restricted and high fiber diet adequate in fruits and vegetables may be taken.

For hypertensive patients, intake of fats- saturated fat may be restricted (like butter, ghee and coconut oil), salt intake should be checked. Foods which contain high amounts of salt should be avoided. Physical activity and maintenance of desirable body weight is must. Eggs, red meat, alcohol and smoking is to be avoided.

As revealed by our studies on local elderly population nutritional status of elderly improved after treating their dental problems. However, it was also seen that there was highly significant decline in taste sensitivity with advancing age and addiction with tobacco and smoking.

Studies also show that age related impairment of the dentition was responsible for decline in masticating efficiency. There were significant changes in the diets of subjects with tooth loss or oral problems. Due to change in food consistency, majority subjects reported loss of appetite, weight loss and food aversions. All these studies reported much lower nutrient intake in edentulous patients or patients with partial teeth loss (Mehta and Panchal 2005). It is recommended that oral problems of the elderly should be attended immediately to avoid health complications.

Generally, edentulous patients may be given blend soft gruels full of energy, carbohydrates and proteins and sufficiently enriched with minerals and vitamins. Soft cooked foods may be included. Sprouting and fermentation process causes ease in digestion. Cooking practices which ease the digestion, help in producing more saliva and facilitate mastication and swallowing may be used. Use of cutlery should be discrete and should not hurt the mouth cavity. Thus, soft and blend cooked foods, mashed or blendarised foods and fruits should be the basic items in diets of elderly with oral cavity problems.

Elderly patients with swallowing disorders also have compromised diets and suffer from multi micronutrient deficiency. In this regards author's team has carried out few studies on such patients with swallowing problems/head and neck cancer (Mehta and Srivastava, 1997). These studies showed that their diets could hardly supply 50 per cent of RDA with regard to important nutrients. Use of household technology was tried out in making the gruels for their feeding trials. Long term feeding trials showed very encouraging results.

All these studies showed that use of ARF technology or fermentation offer better option for modification in consistency and nutrient availability as these types of modification do not involve dilution of Food/gruel but helps in improving food intake at a sitting in patients who cannot swallow solid food.

Nutritional Disorders in Elderly

Ageing brings about progressive loss of tissue function along with the occurrence of chronic diseases.

Osteoporosis is one of such diseases which causes disability in elderly population. Few risk factors such as early menopause, mobilization, life style factors and present as well as past (20–30 yrs of age) dietary calcium intake have been found to be linked with the occurrence of osteoporosis (Patel D and Mehta P., 1999) our studies have also revealed that frequent consumption of certain calcium rich foods in past (during 20–30 years of age) is beneficial. Association of sedentary lifestyle, smoking and use of alcohol, had adverse effect on the development of osteoporosis. Thus, there is need to modify life style factors and dietary practices as early as possible.

The other major chronic degenerative disorder commonly encountered in old age is osteoarthritis. It is pathologically and radiologically defined by reduced joint space and secondary to loss of cartilage by sclerosis of subchondral bone and by osteophyte formations. Weight reduction and exercise play important role in reducing pain and delay functional impairment. This is where diet also plays important role. Author's group (Mehta and Hardasini, 1999) studied 40 overweight osteoporotic women with clinical and radiological signs. The study found significant differences

($P<0.05$) between fat and energy intake and time spent in moderate activities by obese arthritic patients and the control group when odds ratio was applied to study association between dietary factors and occurrence of disease, consumption of nuts and oil seeds, non-veg foods and fried foods were strongly related to occurrence. Frequent consumption of green leafy vegetables (OR = 0.74) and fruits rich in beta carotene and vitamin C (OR = 0.71) was also frequently associated.

After intervention with weight reduction dietary regimen and exercise for 3 months, reduction of pain score units was observed by 3.2 per cent.

Thus, apart from non - dietary factors development of osteoarthritis is also related to dietary factors. Certain food habits like consumption of high fat sweets, nuts and oilseeds, fried items and non-vegetarian foods seem to contribute to the development of osteoarthritis.

Prevalence of anemia in older individuals is about 50 per cent in developed countries and 12 per cent in developing countries (WHO, 2000). Iron deficiency anemia is the second most common cause of anemia in elderly. Our studies conducted earlier (Swati Parnami, Komal Chauhan and Pallavi Mehta, 2005) showed poor dietary intake of iron and decline in physical performance and cognitive function. However, iron folic acid supplementation (325 mg iron sulfate) for 6 weeks showed significant improvement in their anemia status, physical performance and cognitive functions.

Constipation is also one of the commonest complaints from elderly people. Constipation in the elderly may be due to combined causes such as low fiber diet, inadequate fluid, lack of exercise, poor muscle tone, drugs and diseases.

Treatment includes high intake of fluid (2 to 3 litres/ day), regular exercise, high fiber diet/high residue diet and storage avoidance of medicines causing constipation.

Some useful information related to diet in specific condition has been given in a tool used for training caregivers elsewhere in this book.

A wholesome diet with liberal substitutes should be planned for the elderly with 4–5 small needs at fixed intervals. Health and disease conditions and biochemical abnormalities may be taken into account while planning the diet. Weight should be maintained within permissible range & elderly should be encouraged to undergo or yearly medical check up to avoid nutritional problems.

References

Chauhan K and Mehta P (2007), Health Promotion for the aged through intervention with suitable food and nutrient supplementation, PhD. Dissertation (unpublished), Dept. of Foods and Nutrition, The M.S.University, Baroda, Vadodara, India.

Chhabra S and Mehta P (2001), A study on nutritional status, diet and disease profile of edentulous elderly subjects (with and without denture treatment), M.Sc. Dissertation (unpublished), Dept. of Foods and Nutrition, The M.S.University, Baroda, Vadodara, India.

Dhapola P and Mehta P. (2009), Development and evaluation of 'Quick Cooking Food Mix' as a base for Geriatric Feed: Impact evaluation on health and nutritional Status of elderly Subjects, M.Sc. Dissertation (unpublished), Dept. of Foods and Nutrition, the M.S. University, Vadodara, India.

Mehta P and Hardasmi M (1999), A Study on Assessment of nutritional Status, Life Style factors, diet profile and impact of NHE on Osteoarthritic Women (age 50 yrs +) Unpublished M.Sc. dissertation, Dept of Foods and Nutrition, the M.S. University of Baroda, Vadodara, India.

Mehta P and Mehta M (2003), A Study on Nutrition and Disease Profile of Elderly Belonging to three Different Communities, Indian Journal of Gerontology; 17(3 and 4): 380-388

Mehta P and Srivastava R. (1997), Effect of Modified diet on health and nutritional status of Hospitalised male geriatrics (60-70 years) with the swallowing disorders, Unpublished M.Sc. Dissertation, Dept of Foods and Nutrition, The M.S. University of Baroda, Vadodara, India.

Mehta P, Chauhan K and Devi C (2007), Study on food preferences and taste sensitivity of 20–29local elderly women residing in Baroda city and evaluation of selected food items for geriatric group, Indian Journal of Gerontology; 21(1): 20-2921.

Mehta P, Sheth M, Vyas M (1997), Socio-demographic, Nutrition and Health profile of Indian elderlies (50-70 years) living in urban Baroda, India "Reaching the unreached", Department of Foods and Nutrition, The M.S University of Baroda, Vadodara, India.

Mehta P., Sharma M and Chauhan K (2010), A study on health and nutritional status of very old elderly (85 + years) and centenarians, Indian Journal of Gerentology, Vol. 23, No. 2: 277-284.

Parnami S, Chauhan K and Mehta P (2005), A study on nutrition, diet and disease profile of the elderly anemic women with or without intervention through iron folic acid supplementation, Indian journal of gerontology; 19(2): 147-156.

Patel D and Mehta P (1999), A study on lifestyle factors, nutritional status and Dietary profile of women and men in relation to osteoporotic fractures: NHEprogram as a strategy for prevention (age 50 years onwards) M.Sc. Dissertation (unpublished), Dept. of Foods and Nutrition, The M.S. University, Baroda, Vadodara, India.

Patil G and Chauhan K (2007), A study on nutritional and health profile of depressed elderly women of Baroda city: Impact of herbal intervention with Ashwagandha (Withaniasomnifera) on mental health of elderly women M.Sc. Dissertation (unpublished), Dept. of Foods and Nutrition, The M.S. University, Baroda, Vadodara, India.

Vasavda T and Mehta P (2003), A study on Assessment of Diet, Nutrition and Health Profile of Elderly (Aged 60 yrs and above) in religious order, Indian Journal of Gerontology; 17(3 and 4): 389-397.

6

Suitable Foods for Geriatric Feeding

"We eat to live and not live to eat. Good diet is a perfect way of curing and worthy much regard to health assuring."

–Unknown

Malnutrition amongst elderly is a growing problem. In reality the fastest growing segment of the population in most industrialised countries is the elderly and too often this is also a group most susceptible to many health risks because of nutrient poor diets. Evidence from numerous sources indicate that significant number of elderly fail to get the amounts and types of food necessary to meet essential energy and nutrients needs. Infact, as mentioned in earlier chapter's author's team has consistently shown lower food intake in elderly since past two and half decades in series of studies undertaken by them. As the individual ages, there are many metabolic and physiological changes which show an impact on the nutritional needs of an individual. Even with a increased calorie need, many people have difficulty in getting sufficient calories which can eventually lead to chronic fatigue, depression and a weakened immune system.

With ageing the body composition changes with a decrease in lean body mass (as much as 25 per cent) and an increase in body fat. Such changes can be accelerated because older adults utilise dietary protein less efficiently and may actually need a greater then recommended amount of high quality protein in their diet to maintain lean body mass. These changes in metabolism and physiology can be exaggerated due to complication from digestive difficulties, oral and dental problems and medication related eating and nutrient problems.

Many can contribute to under nutrition in the elderly. There are also many equally important social and economic factors, which can further complicate the nutritional well-being of an older individual. Contributing factors include loneliness, lack of cooking skills, depression, economic concerns, weakness and fatigue and in many cases an unwarranted fear of using much high quality, nutrient dense, unaffordable food. All these factors can contribute to the fact that a significant number of older men and women consume less food then required to meet energy and nutrient requirements and are at moderate to high nutritional deficiency risk.

Arthritis makes it difficult for the elderly living alone to shop for and prepare food. Decreased activity to taste and smell can also affect the enjoyment of food. For the elderly, poor dentition, loss of teeth and poor fitted dentures cause chewing problems and mouth sores making eating process difficult.

Those living alone and who face financial difficulties tend to skip on food and many cook only one dish a day to be eaten over breakfast, lunch and dinner. Many elderly men (after the death of their spouse) neglect their nutrition because they lack the cooking skills and knowledge of nutrition and suffer from problems such as loneliness, depression or weakness and fatigue. Others eat too much of fatty foods or deep fried foods instead of nutrient dense foods like fruits, vegetables, whole grains (Health promotion board, 2001).

The nutritional risk of the elderly is also affected by the fact that low fat, low cholesterol diet message has been heard loud and clear by this population. Many elderly readily accept the fear of consuming high fat and cholesterol diet because of their heightened concern regarding their own health and the knowledge that the risk for chronic diseases increases with age, while dietary limits on fat and cholesterol consumption are widely assumed to be effective risk reduction interventions in young and middle aged adult, the appropriateness of such dietary restrictions in older individuals has become an area of considerable debate,

Good nutrition is requirement for all ages and more so for older people as quality of their diet is basic to the quality of their life. Many older individuals lack nutrition balance as there is over emphasis on single nutrient issues.

Dietary Problems Leading to Food Inadequacy in Elderly

Some elderly individuals encounter dietary problems, making them less able to select, purchase, prepare, eat, digest, absorb and use food. It is important to intervene to correct any dietary problem that may exist. Dietary problems and interventions to solve these problems are discussed here.

(a) Difficulty in Chewing or Swallowing

Loss of teeth and high rate of dental problems in the elderly causes difficulty in chewing and swallowing of foods. One of the studies carried out by our team showed that elderly patients who had oral cavity problems like chewing and swallowing had very poor nutritional status. To overcome this problem, gruel was prepared using Amylase Rich Food (ARF) technology, where in cereal is sprouted, dried and powdered. When ten per cent of this powder was used to prepare the gruel/porridge, did not change the consistency on cooling. Therefore further results showed that patients could eat approximately 120 ml more food than before with improvement in their well-being and nutritional status at the end of 6 weeks of intervention program (Shrivastava and Mehta, 1997). On the other hand same type of gruel was also fed to elderly suffering from head and neck cancer. Remarkable improvement in health and nutritional status with reduction of hospital stay was reported (Chhabra and Mehta, 2000).

Dhapola et al., 2009, prepared such gruel as a base food using ARF prepared out of ragi and fed to institutionalised elderly largely having denture problems in the morning not only improved their physical health (weight, activities) but also benefitted mental health with regard to MMSE and CIT scores.

In order to overcome dietary inadequacy due to chewing problems, one can choose milk, fruits and vegetable juices, soft canned fruits, creamed or mashed cooked vegetables, eggs, milk dishes, soups, cheese, yogurt and cooked cereals, combination of cereal and pulses like khichadi, boiled dals with or without addition of cooked vegetables. One can grate, stew, chop or steam hard foods.

For difficult situations like presence of swallowing disorders such as head and neck cancers, maintenance of good nutritional status often becomes a problem. Pallavi Mehta and Manimala Mandapati (1997), conducted trials with dietary modifications which included the use of ARF (Amylase Rich Food) in preparation of wheat flour based gruel at 20 per cent concentration with 5 gm addition of ARF. ARF from wheat grain was prepared by steeping, germination, oven drying, devegetation and milling. When this gruel was fed for one month to control and experimental group, with and without addition of ARF, experimental group had gruel intake with ARF showed 59 per cent greater gruel consumption and improvement in general health at the end of one month than control group fed only gruel without ARF.

In another study done by Pallavi Mehta and Radhika Shrivastav (1997) on fifty patients with swallowing difficulty other than cancer, dietary nutrient intake was reported to be less then recommended dietary allowances (RDA). Dietary modification was carried out using fermented cereal pulse gruel to which 5 gm ARF was added to adjust the viscosity processed and unprocessed gruels were fed for three days each separately to the hospitalised elderly subjects with swallowing disorder for a period of 7 weeks. There was 41 per cent increase in the intake of processed gruel as compared to unprocessed gruel with improvement in general health and nutritional status.

Both the above studies suggest scope of using malting and fermentation technology for geriatric feeding for therapeutic purpose as well as hospital setting.

(b) Difficulty in Digesting

Decrease in the secretion of digestive juices, dental and gastro intestinal tract related problems lead to difficulty in digesting foods. To solve this problem one must select fruits and vegetable juices, non gas forming vegetables and well cooked cereals. Among pulses, moong dal (green gram dal) seems to be the best. Curd and buttermilk can also be included. Germinated cereals and legumes and fermented cereals and legumes are good alternative to diets as there is also decrease in the flatulence factor.

(c) Decrease in Appetite

Lack of physical activity, decreased gastric tone. Diminished secretion of gastric juices and too many medications are the major contributory factors for decreased appetite for an elderly living in normal environment. Variety in food, pleasant atmosphere, good company and mild flavour of spices and herbs can keep the elderly to increase food intake.

(d) Difficulty in Shopping and Cooking

Shopping related activities like counting money, walking in crowded area, crossing the roads etc. may lead to avoidance of such activities resulting in compromise with food intake.

Help through paid volunteers or shopping through phone or "Home health services" may be suggested.

Arthritis, problem in standing position or bending may make elaborate cooking procedures difficult task for elderly. Simple easy to make nutrition preparation can make the life easy for elderly home makers.

In this connection, result obtained by author's study conducted on elderly women with different living arrangements on problems related to food activity are worth noting (Chauhan K. and Mehta P. 2007).

(e) Social Problems

Loneliness while eating and living alone and both correlated with lower quality diets. Man may be at greater risk because they are less experienced with planning, shopping and preparing meals. Women may feel less motivated to prepare meals when there is no one to share with. Ways to improve social interaction during meals and improve the experience of dinning alone include: participating with them and congregate dinning sites, eating by window, eating in a park or inviting friends/family occasionally.

When health of elderly is changed by living alone, possibility of adult day care, in home care, retirement communities, residential care or assisted living and old age nursing homes may be considered.

(f) Medical, Physical and Functional Problems

Many chronic medical conditions such as osteoporosis, depression, diabetes and some deliberating disorders have nutritional consequences. At times, specialised diets or medical nutrition therapy are needed. There are many elderly who need special diets but are not able to follow the regime due to difficulty or inconvenience in preparation or procurement of foods suitable for them.

Many a times when an individual reaches a particular age, the sense of taste deteriorates, which can result in potentially dangerous conditions such as malnourishment or susceptibility to disease. This may affect both physical and mental health of many elderly people.

For improving the nutritional status of the elderly, as a first step exercise may be a good way to increase muscle strength and control blood sugar levels. Regularity in eating meal at prospective and modifying of food as per body need will definitely help. Eating with friends or dine out in public on some days may help in breaking monotony of diet and avoidance of isolation. Caregiver can ascertain that crunch and colour is added to the diet and there is new variety to try for elderly. A glass of water may be required along with meals. Even food items should include lot of fluid based material. Taking two or three bites of food and switching over to another may help in getting variety of flavours and textures.

Studies by Jong et al., 2001, showed beneficial effects of interventions with nutrient dense foods, exercise or combination of both in free living frail elderly.

Variety and assortment are important compartments of healthful diet.

Home helpers services can be sought if necessary. However, a home helper should not take over completely but facilitate procedure so that the elderly can manage as long as possible (Andersson and Sidenvall, 2001).

Food related health promotion must pay more attention to elderly living alone. Women who have lost their partners may be at risk for poor nutritional intake as they often simplified the meal situation, while collating women perceived food and cooking as a central task in their lives (Gustafsson and Sidervall, 2002).

Looking into the food related problems faced by the elderly in different situation and with different living arrangement; a study was conducted in author's laboratory where few items were formulated using soybean (category A) and few items requiring minimum cooking (category B) suitable for geriatric feeding. Category A included four soya based items. Category B included vegetable and milk based quick cooking items. Soya items were developed that it contained 17–23 gms of soya protein. Nutritive composition of soy based items are given below.

Sr. No	Food Items	Protein (gms) Mean ± SD		% RDA	Fat (gms) Mean ± SD		% RDA
1.	Soy Based	Calculated Values	Analyzed Values		Calculated Values	Analyzed Values	
a.	**Soy usal**	15.17	12.70 ± 0.14	25	17.02	17.00 ± 0.94	56.6
b.	Soy sambhar	12.57	10.73 ± 0.89	21.5	10.50	8.35 ± 0.38	27.8
c.	Soy dhokli	12.72	10.43 ± 0.86	21	15.15	14.41 ± 3.86	48
d.	Soy stuffed paratha	14.15	11.78 ± 0.3	24	10.33	7.08 ± 0.5	23.6
e.	Soy roti	6.08	5.90 ± 0.07	12	5.45	5.26 ± 0.28	17.5
2.	**Quick**						
a.	Carrot kheer	4.30	3.99 ± 0.87	8	1.32	1.03 ± 0.1	3.4
b.	Spinach in white sauce	6.03	5.85 ± 0.12	12	2.96	2.06 ± 1.42	6.8

Items were subjected to sensory evaluation by a panel of trained judges (n=21) using Hedonic scale. Evaluation was also carried out by elderly themselves (free living as well as institutionalised). All items received high acceptability scores (See figure below).

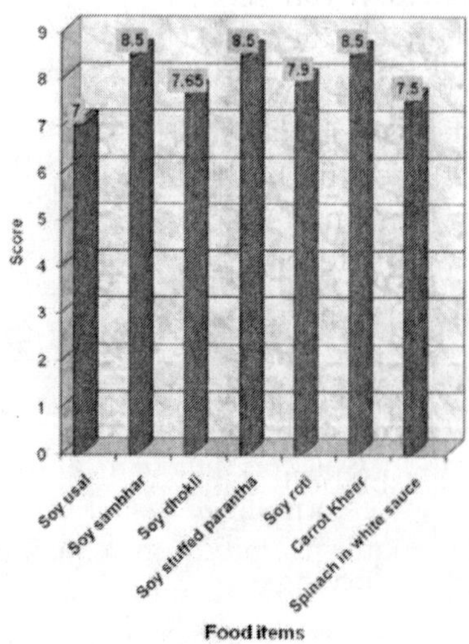

Fig. I. Mean scores of various food items on a 9-point Hedonic scale.

The same study was extended further to assess the beneficial effect of soya foods on health and nutritional status of institutionalised elderly subjects.

For this purpose 20 occupants of PremdasJalaramVridh Ashram were daily supplied soya items for breakfast and soya roti for meals, which contained 14-23gm of soya protein per day as partial supplement for 3 months.

Post intervention data showed significant increase in body weight ($p<0.05$). Nutrient intake also improved significantly reaching 100 per cent of RDA for most of the nutrients.

There was significant improvement in clinical parameters like haemoglobin and LDL cholesterol and HDL cholesterol ($p<0.05$). Blood glucose levels and blood pressure levels were also reduced to normal after intervention. It was worth noting that fifty per cent of the elderly subjects showed reduction in number and severity of minor illnesses after intervention with soya foods for 3 months.

Thus, the study showed that intervention with food or nutrient supplementation can serve as an effective strategy for promoting health for the aged.

In one study by Mehta et al., 2010, nutritional status, signs of ageing, disease profile, food preferences and taste sensitivity were studied in 140 elderly in Vadodara city. Formulation and evaluation of selected food items was carried out based on their preferences.

Based on the preferences of elderly, five food items were standardised in the laboratory and evaluated using composite testing by trained panel members and the elderly population. The five different food items were: Green paratha, stuffed vegetable idli, daliakhichadi, soybean puda and soybean puranpoli.

Green Paratha: (2 servings)

Ingredients	**Amounts**
Wheat flour	70 g

Gram flour	20 g
Soya flour	20 g
Green gram sprouts	25 g
Spinach	25 g
Carrots	25 g
Onion	50 g
Green chilly	1 no.
Butter	1 tsp.
Salt to taste	

Procedure

- Grind the sprouts and grate the carrots.
- Chop the onion, green chilly and spinach.
- Mix wheat flour, gram flour and soya flour and add salt to it.
- Mix the sprouts, grated carrots and the chopped onions and green chilly to the flour and prepare a smooth dough out of it.
- Make small balls of the dough and roll out the chappaties.

Nutrient Composition Per Serving

Energy	:	269 Kcal
Carbohydrate	:	40.96 gm
Protein	:	13.91 gm
Fat	:	5.37 gm

Stuffed Vegetable Idli: (4 Servings)

For Batter:

Ingredients	**Amounts**
Semolina	150 g
Rice flakes	45 g
Urad dal	45 g
Salt	to taste

For Stuffing:

Ingredients	**Amounts**
Carrot	60 g
Capsicum	25 g
Green peas	100 g
Green chilies	2 nos.
Curry leaves	3–4 nos.
Mustard seeds	½ tsp.
Urad dal	½ tsp.
Oil	¼ tsp.

Procedure:

For Batter:

% Soak the semolina and rice flakes for 2 hours.

% Soak urad dal separately for 2 hours.

% Grind semolina and rice flakes to a fine paste in a grinder.

% Grind urad dal separately.

% Mix both the pastes and add salt to taste.

For Stuffing:

- Grind all the vegetables in a grinder.
- Heat ¼ tsp oil in a pan, add mustard seeds, curry leaves and green chilies.
- Add the vegetables and fry for 3–4 minutes.
- Mix this stuffing with the batter and steam in an idli stand for 10–15 minutes.
- Serve hot with coconut chutney.

Nutrient Composition Per Serving

Energy	: 221 Kcal
Carbohydrate	: 46.05 gm
Protein	: 4.48 gm

Fat : 0.5 gm

Dahlia Khichdi: (4 Servings)

Ingredients	**Amounts**
Dahlia	1 cup
Roasted & finely powdered groundnuts	½ cup
Cumin powder	1 tsp
Coriander leaves minced	20 g
Green chilies minced	3 nos.
Carrot minced	40 g
Bottle gourd minced	40 g
Paneer mashed	50 g
Soya bean oil	5 Tbsp
Salt to taste	

Procedure:

- Wash and drain the dahlia.
- Heat 5 Tbsp oil and add the masala, fry for some time and add the rest of the ingredients.
- Add water, cover and cook over a slow fire till done.

Nutrient Composition Per Serving:

Energy :	664.82 Kcal
Carbohydrate :	44.83 gm
Protein :	56.65 gm
Fat :	40.46 gm

Soya – besan Puda: (2 Servings)

Ingredients	**Amounts**
Gram flour	50 g
Soya flour	50 g
Red chilly powder	¼ tsp
Coriander powder	¼ tsp
Cumin powder	¼ tsp

Turmeric powder	½ tsp
Ajwain, whole	½ tsp
White sesame seeds	½ tsp
Oil	35 ml
Water	220 ml
Salt to taste	

Procedure:

- Mix the gram flour with the soya flour.
- Add all the spices, sesame seeds and salt into the flour mixture and mix well.
- Add water and make a smooth batter.
- Heat a flat non-stick griddle and smear it lightly with oil.
- Pour the batter with a ladle and spread it thinly on the griddle into a circular shape.
- Take a little oil in a teaspoon and pour it around the edge to make it crisp.
- When the batter is set turn it over with a pancake turner.
- Slit it off the griddle after a minute.

Nutrient Composition Per Serving:

Energy :	371.82 Kcal
Carbohydrate :	20.37 gm
Protein :	16.8 gm
Fat :	24.75 gm

Soya bean Puranpoli: (2 Servings)

Ingredients	Amounts
Soyabeans	80 g
Red gram dal	20 g
Soyabean flour	40 g
Wheat flour	160 g

Sugar	150 g
Oil	50 g
Cardamom powder	10 g

Procedure:

- Soak the soyabeans and the red gram dal separately overnight.
- Dehusk the soyabeans.
- Prepare a dough out of the soyabean flour and wheat flour.
- Boil the soyabeans and the red gram dal in just adequate amount of water.
- Blend the pulses in a mixture grinder along with the sugar and cardamom powder.
- Heat this mixture on a hot iron griddle by constantly stirring until it thickens into a consistency equal to the dough and divide them into small equal sized balls.
- Roll out small chappaties and stuff into them these balls and roll them again.
- Shallow fry these on a flat frying pan with just adequate amount of oil.

Nutrient Composition Per Serving:

Energy :	1089 Kcal
Carbohydrate:	148.39 gm
Protein :	37.9 gm
Fat :	38.24 gm

All items were found to be acceptable by elderly. When asked about the preferences of each item for a particular meal, dalia khichadi and green paratha were mostly preferred for breakfast by elderly as age advance. Stuffed vegetable idli, soybean puda and soybean puranpoli were maximum preferred for tea time by all elderly subjects. Elderly subjects from 50-70 years and 71-85 years old groups preferred to consume full katori of dalia khichadi. Green paratha and soybean puranpoli were preferred in lesser amount by older subjects (8.6 per cent). However, soybean puda was preferred in more amounts by the young olds and old olds.

The finding of the study suggested that food preferences and food intake are affected by advancement of age. Taste sensitivity seems to be affected after fifth decade but changes are well marked in seventh decade. The elderly preferred food items that were easy to chew and were softer.

Development of food products with functional properties for geriatric group was also attempted to study the effect on health by author's research team of Foods and Nutrition dept. at M.S. University of Baroda (Mehta et al., 2010). The product studied were Ragiladoo/Ragiladoo and Amladrink and Ragiladdoo and Shankhapushpi (Unjha Co. make syrup was used). The developed food products were subjected to acceptability trials and met 1/3rd RDA of elderly for energy, protein, fibre, iron and calcium. Products were fed for five weeks to eighty elderly subjects belonging to two old age institutions of Vadodara city. Assessment after post intervention included assessment of nutritional status, disease profile and mental and physical health status.

Table I. Nutritive value of Ragiladoo per serving (2 ladoos)

Ingredients	*Amount(gm)*	*Protein(gm)*	*Fat (gm)*	*Fiber (gm)*	*Energy (Kcal)*	*Calcium (mg)*	*Iron (mg)*
Ragi flour	50	3.6	0.65	1.8	164	172	1.95
Soyabean flour	15	6.48	2.92	0.5	65	36	1.56
Niger seeds	10	2.4	3.88	1.09	52	30	5.67
Ghee	20	-	20	-	180	-	-
Jaggery	37	0.14	0.03	-	142	30	1
Total	132	12.62	27.4	3.4	603	268	10.18

Table II. Nutritive value of Amla Drink per serving

Ingredients	*Amount (gm/ml)*	*Energy (Kcal)*	*Vitamin C (mg)*	*Fiber (gm)*
Amla powder	10	6	19.2	1.5
Sugar	5	20	-	-
Sugar free natura	0.5	0.12	-	-
Water	100	-	-	-
Total		26	19.2	1.5

Beneficial effects of supplementation of Ragiladoo on subjects was seen with regard to weight gain, lipid profile and dietary intake. The prevalence of minor illnesses reduced and the overall physical performance improved satisfactorily.

The group of subjects supplemented with Ragi ladoo and Amla juice/Shankhpushpi showed weight gain, improvement in dietary intake. The MMSE scores showing cognitive function improved ($P<0.05$) significantly. Grip strength and timed physical activities also showed positive change.

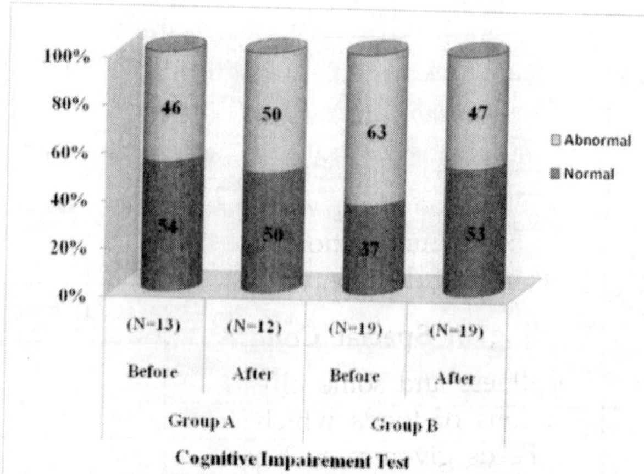

Fig. II: Percentage of elderly subject showing cognitive power as per CIT score before and after intervention (Group A Ladoo and Group B Ladoo+Shankhpushpi)

Table III: Percentage of elderly subjects from both groups, falling under various categories of GDI, MMSE and CIT before and after the intervention

Mental Health	*Group 1 (Ladoo)*		*Group 2 (Ladoo+drink)*	
	Before Intervention (N=13)	*After Intervention (N=12)*	*Before Intervention (N=20)*	*After Int ervention (N=20)*
GDI				
Normal (0-10)	61.5 (8)	61.5 (8)	50 (10)	45 (9)
Mild (11-15)	38.4 (5)	33.3 (4)	10 (2)	20 (4)
Moderate (16-20)	0 (0)	0 (0)	30 (6)	30 (6)
Severe (>20)	0 (0)	0 (0)	10 (2)	5 (1)
MMSE				
Severe ($\leq$10)	0 (0)	0 (0)	5 (1)	0 (0)
Moderate (11-20)	53.8 (7)	58.3 (7)	40 (8)	25 (5)
Mild (21-26)	30.7 (4)	33.3 (4)	25 (5)	35 (7)
Normal (>26)	15.3 (2)	8.3 (1)	30 (6)	40 (8)
CIT				
Normal (0-10)	58.8 (7)	50 (6)	65 (13)	65 (13)
Abnormal (11-28)	46.1 (6)	50 (6)	35 (7)	35 (7)

Figures in parenthesis denote the total number of subjects

Thus, these studies indicated good acceptability by elderly and beneficial effect on them with respect to physical and mental health. Food intervention of this kind of functional foods can be a successful strategy to improve geriatric health.

Geriatric Feeding in Special Conditions

In case of illness and some physical conditions demand extra specifications of foods which make geriatric feeding little difficult. Feeds given to such patients need to be easy to swallow, easy to digest and should supply greater amount of nutrients at a sitting or ensure more consumption of food at a stretch. Both ways could improve the nutritional status which is crucial for surgical procedures or for disease recovery.

The management of geriatric feeding in hospital setting is often challenging and important job. As such, food intake is inadequate in elderlies and much more inadequate among hospitalised elderly. Some chewing and swallowing disorders need great attention as these conditions can further limit their food intake. A major factor in swallowing of food is consistency. Two major technologies used for reducing viscosity and improving consistency are amylase rich food preparation (ARF) and fermentation.

In this connection, a couple of studies conducted by authors and their co workers are worth noting (Mehta P, Mandapati M and Srivastava R, (2001).

In one study modification using wheat based gruel with Amylase Rich Food was tried out on geriatric patients of ENT Department of S S G Hospital, Vadodara, who were suffering from swallowing disorders. For this purpose, wheat based gruel was prepared at 20 per cent concentration with 5 gm addition of ARF. ARF from wheat grain was prepared by steeping, germination, oven drying, de-vegetation and milling. Consistent viscosity reduction was observed with addition of ARF measured by Brookefield's viscometer. This ARF was added to gruels and fed to elderly for one month. Improvement in gruel intake was found in patients fed with ARF added gruel as compared to patients fed with plain gruels. There was no deterioration in health and slight improvement in body weight and haemoglobin was noted.

The study showed clearly that the use of ARF technology may find place in geriatric clinics and ENT wards having patients with swallowing problems.

The second study included the introduction and the intervention with fermented gruel with addition of ARF to hospitalised elderly (n=15) with swallowing disorder, for seven weeks. Findings showed positive effect on nutrient intake and ease of preparation of feed.

These studies indicate further scope of developing functional foods for therapeutic purposes for disease like cancer and other NCDs.

Some suggested recipes are mentioned here for the use of geriatric feeding in health and disease.

1. Dalia (Wheat/Oats).
2. Vegetable Upma (Rava/cracked wheat).
3. Vegetable Khichadi (Rice/Cracked Wheat/Oats with and without vegetables).
4. Carrot Halwa/Kheer.
5. Vegetable Paratha (mix veg.).
6. Paneer Paratha (Paneer and mix veg).
7. Vegetable Hotch Potch (Soaked Bajra+Rice+Moong dal + vegetables).
8. Puda with vegetables like spinach, tomato, onion, methi.
9. Vegetable Handwa (Potato covering with vegetable stuffing inside).
10. Stuffed Idlis.
11. Sandwich Dhokla.
12. Pancakes with vegetable filling.
13. Vegetable Chaat.
14. Moong dal dumplings in veg. gravy.
15. Kanki and Veg. Soup.
16. Steamed Muthia with veg. gravy.
17. Dudhio Bajro (soaked bajra with upper covering removed and cooked in milk with sugar. Garnish with elaichi and coconut).
18. Flaxseed chutney powder.
19. Roasted bajra, rice and dal powder (to cook in hot water or buttermilk with veg.).
20. Khajoor pak.

References

Andersson I and Sidenvall B (2001), Case studies of food shopping, cooking and eating habits in older women with Parkinson's disease, Journal of Advanced Nursing, Vol. 35, No. 1: 69.

Chauhan and Mehta (2007), Health promotion for the aged through intervention with suitable foods and nutrient supplementation, unpublished doctorate thesis, Department of Foods and Nutrition, Faculty of Family and Community Sciences, M.S. University of Baroda, Vadodara.

Dey A B (2003), Ageing in India, Rakmo Press Pvt., Ltd., New Delhi.

Gustafsson K and Sidenvall B (2002), Food-related health perceptions and food habits among older women, J of AdvNur, Vol. 39, No. 2: 164–73.

Hardasani M (1999), A study on assessment of nutritional status, lifestyle factors, diet profile and impact of NHE on osteoarthritic women (age 50 years onwards), Unpublished M. Sc dissertation, Department of Foods and Nutrition, Faculty of Home Science, The M.S. University of Baroda, Vadodara.

Health Promotion Board (2001), Health A-Z Online, Nutrition for the elderly, Singapore.

Jong, Nynke De (2001), Nutrient-dense foods and exercise in frail elderly: effects on B vitamins, homocysteine, methylmalonic acid and neuropsychological functioning, Am J ClinNutr, 73: 338-46.

Mehta P (1999), Diet, nutrition and health profile of elderly population of urban Baroda Cited from: Ageing Nutrition and Health, Published by Dept. of Foods and Nutrition, M.S. University, Baroda, 54-60.

Mehta P, Chauhan K and Chayanika Devi (2000), Study on food preferences and taste sensitivity of local elderly women residing in Baroda city and evaluation of selected food items for geriatric group, Ind J of Geron, Vol. 21, No. 1, 20-29.

Mehta P, Chauhan K and Gandhi H (2010), A report on Health Promotion Through Nutritionally Improved Recipes for Feeding Vulnerable Groups, submitted to Gujarat State Forest Development Corporation Limited.

Mehta P and Dhapola P (2009), Development and evaluation of 'Quick cooking food mix' as a base for geriatric feed: Impact evaluation on health and nutritional status of elderly subjects, unpublished masters dissertation thesis, Department of Foods and Nutrition, Faculty of Family and Community Sciences, MS University of Baroda, Vadodara.

Mehta P and Manimala M (1996), A study on dietary modification of Hospitalised elderly with swallowing disorders, Unpublished M.Sc. dissertation, Department of Foods and Nutrition, The M.S. University, Baroda, Vadodara.

Patel D (1999), A study on life style factors, nutritional status and dietary profile of women and men in relation to osteoporotic fractures: NHE program as a strategy for prevention (age 50 years onwards, Unpublished M.Sc. dissertation, Department of Foods and Nutrition, Faculty of Home Science, The M.S.University of Baroda, Vadodara.

Srivastava R and Mehta P (1997), Effect of Modified diet on Health and Nutritional Status of Hospitalised male geriatrics (60-70 yrs.) with the swallowing disorders. Unpublished M.Sc. Dissertion, Dept. of Foods and Nutrition, The M.S. University of Baroda, Vadodara, India.

Vasavda T and Mehta P., (2003), A study on Assessment of Diet, Nutriton and Health Profile of Elderly (Aged 60 yrs and above) in religious order Indian Journal of Gerontology; 17(3 and 4): 389-397.

7

Caregiving: Emerging Need of Elderly Today

'The joy of loving is the joy of sharing, so let us share the joy of loving by helping each other, to help the people who need love'.

–Mother Teressa

Ageing is associated with a decline in physical and mental health. As the population age is rectangularised, there is a growing concern in Asia with how the elderly will be supported and cared in the twenty first century. Rapid urbanization has resulted in breaking up of the traditional joint family system. Even in joint families, the health and nutritional status of the elderly depends on the caregivers to a large extent. According to national long term care survey (1994), more than seven million persons are informal caregivers mainly women as a daughter in law, wife, daughter, etc. and provide unpaid help to older persons who live in the community and have at least one limitation in their activities of daily living. In the family there is usually one primary caregiver – a role traditionally held by a women.

The typical profile of a today's female caregiver is that of middle aged individual between the ages of 40 and 60 years with two to three children who may still be living at home and who also may demand her attention and care.

In a study by Sharma (1998) in South India, it was reported that for 94 per cent elderly men, source of care during sickness was either by spouses, unmarried children or sons. On the other hand for elderly women, the source of such care sons (50 per cent) and daughter was (28 per cent). The care provided by spouses was limited to only 3 per cent.

Family support is an important factor for better psychological well-being. Lack of caregiver is a serious problem for those older persons who have chronic condition and limitations on their ability to care for themselves and their homes. Their problems are often compounded by increased medical cost due to poor health and the need for more supportive services.

Why are problems of caregiving on increase?

- In most traditional societies, the family provides care to in older members various socioeconomic and cultural changes such as the strain on the joint family system have disrupted this age old set up by increasing burden of caregiving.
- People are now living longer and this has increased the number of generation living together.
- Housing being very expensive and living space being small, accommodating several generations of old people is becoming harder. This is especially true if the older person requires an aid such as walker or a wheel chair.
- Traditionally, women usually the daughters in law and sometimes daughters have been responsible for the care of the elderly. For economic reasons, more and more women are going outside the home for work. As a result, the traditional care model is getting disrupted.

- Long term care of a frail and physically dependent older person leads to variety of physical, emotional, social and financial stresses for the caregiver (Dey, 2003).

Increased caregiver burden relates to decreased mental and physical health. Apart from providing good care, a care provider should aim at helping elderly individuals to cope more effectively with the stresses of illness or disability enhance their feelings of self worth and value, comply with prescribed medical regimen and if possible, make a speedy recovery from illness or diseases.

Care of the carer is also very vital issue which is often neglected in Indian families. The caregiver is usually the "hidden patient" and the health worker or other family members should pay attention to the needs of the caregiver. Prolonged stress of caring indirectly affects the well-being and living condition of older person. This may at times lead to abuse or neglect of the elderly.

Advancing age brings about various problems which interferes in the day to day routine activities of the elderly. These problems can be with respect to reduced mobility, diminished vision along with other physical and functional impairments. All these problems affect the health of elderly resulting in increased demands for caregiving. Looking at the current scenario regarding health profile of elderly subjects, it is apparent that in the coming years, burden of disease and disability in elderly will increase with the increase in their population. Caring for disabled or dependent elderly family members is strenuous and is difficult to attend to in today's fast paced world. Prasad and Rani (2007) conducted a study on home caregivers of elderly in India and found that caregivers from nuclear households reported higher burdens compared to joint or extended household.

Caring for elderly patients is a very demanding job which require great deal of skill and patience. Moremoto et al. (2003) conducted a study in Japan on 100 family caregivers of elderly stroke patients and found that the caregivers were depressed owing to the stress of caregiving. Prevalence of depression in caregiver was found to be twice as that in the elderly care recipients.

On the other hand, there is a need for capacity building of caregivers of the elderly and sensitise caregivers and other family members towards the special needs of elderly.

Caregiving requires immense understanding and ability to keep cool and level headed at all times.

Home Care and Self-caregiving

There are many factors which determine ageing and which can be controlled by proper care. Nutrition is the most important factor which affects the health of the elderly. Due to increase in the life expectancy along with newer problems of health care, financial constraints and disease due to changed life styles have predisposed the elderly population at the risk of under nutrition. This burden of under nutrition further adds to the challenges for the home caregivers. One of the reasons for poor nutritional status of elderly is poor knowledge of home caregivers. A study carried out to assess the role of antioxidants on health and diseases during ageing process on 166 men and women (45 yrs and above) reported that the caregivers were ignorant about various physiological changes, disorders occurring with advancing age and relationship between diet and degenerative diseases. The data also indicated that very few caregivers of the elderly were found to put the knowledge into action (Mehta and Shringarpure, 2004). It may be noted that authors research team has conducted several studies in past on lifestyle pattern, diet, nutrition and disease profile of the elderly and reported that nutrient intake in most of the elderly was below RDA except for fat. This finding has been consistant in all her studies conducted so far (1991 to 2010).

Our society has traditionally treated the care of the elderly as the responsibility of the younger generation. However, the rapid increase in the number of nuclear families, growing urbanization and the global nature of employment opportunities are forcing a change in this implicit social contract. These challenges are compelling many of our elderly to live alone. Most of them resort to self-care.

Self-care has long been recognised as the major facet of health care and has been defined as the decisions and actions individuals take with regard to their own health self-care be considered as an important determinant of health, concerned with the development and use of personal health practices and coping skills.

A study carried out by western green et al. (2002) in Sweden on 144 male and female elderly patients (> 70 yrs) suggested that elderly patients who perceived good health had higher self-care ability and stronger sense of coherence than patients who perceived ill health.

The existing knowledge of the self-caregiver elderly with respect to dietary care, self-care and health needs of the elderly determines the awareness regarding various aspects of ageing. Elderly who are living alone are ignorant about their health. Providing older persons with information about their own health situation and what they can do about it may facilitate self-care capacity building interventions.

Nutrition Health Education interventions are intended to encourage long term adoption of healthful eating patterns in free living population. Increasing evidences indicated that such interventions can be appealing and effective means of improving nutrition.

In this connection studies conducted by Panchal and Mehta, (2005) showed interesting findings. One of their studies basically focused on assessing the knowledge and practices of caregivers of the elderly (> 75 yrs) and evaluation of impact of Nutrition Health Education (NHE) on knowledge retention and practices of caregivers was also studied.

The baseline data revealed that the mean age of elderly care recipients was < 80 years. More than 82 per cent subjects resided in joint families and half of them were married. In case of caregivers of the elderly mean age was 50 years and were females (Daughter-in-law or wife).

In lower income group, one fourth of the caregivers in elderly population were self-caregiver. The data also revealed that 40 per cent caregivers from HIG and MIG had better perception regarding ageing. Irrespective of economic status majority i.e. more than 78 per cent caregivers were ignorant about minor and major health problems and physiological changes taking place in old age. Nutritional disorders occuring in old age were known to 50 per cent of MIG, HIG group whereas LIG caregivers had poor knowledge about the same. Majority of caregivers (85 per cent) had good knowledge about psychological problems during ageing.

Knowledge regarding dietary aspects in old age was fair to poor in majority of caregivers. This aspect included knowledge regarding number of meals, consistency of food and water requirement. Practices of meal pattern included changes in consumption of foods such as whole grain, whole pulses and unhealthy foods like fried foods and sweet food. Water intake was observed to be very poor in 20–40 per cent of elderly.

Elderly under study had poor disease profile with respect to oral cavity problems (88 per cent) followed by nervous (60 per cent) and GIT problems (64 per cent).

Food frequency data showed that consumption of vitamin c rich foods in males (46.7 per cent) and intake of fiber and fluids in females (80 per cent) had increased after NHE intervention.

Overall health care practices improved after imparting nutritional health intervention. A couple of studies conducted by the geriatric research team of the authors (Mehta and Gupta 2009, Chauhan et al, 2010) aimed at assessing the knowledge and practices of the elderly male and female self-caregivers (≥65 yrs) and building up their capacity as caregivers through Nutrition Health Education (NHE) intervention. These studies had a great relevance to present scenario where there is a social change leading to breakdown of the joint family resulting in increase in numbers of elderly living alone and taking care of themselves alone.

Data on socio demographic and lifestyle factors revealed that majority of male self-caregivers from elder group were 70+ years, married and living with their spouses, spent most of their time in leisure activities and almost $1/4^{th}$ of elderly population under study was found to have some addiction. Similar assessment of female elderly self givers showed mean age of 67 to 75 years in younger and older age group respectively. Older group has 33 per cent of widows and majority of them had received school education and were spending idle time with hardly any activity. Data on nutritional status revealed that female elderly group showed higher prevalence of obesity (62 per cent) whereas most of the older men showed normal BMI. However, prevalence of anemia was very high (81 per cent) in female elderly self-caregivers compared to male elderly self-caregivers (48 per cent) $1/3^{rd}$ of them were diabetic most of the subjects could meet the requirement up to 75- 100 per cent RDA for energy and protein. However, Iron and fibers consumption was very poor in elderly subjects.

Elderly male caregivers though perceived themselves as healthy, showed dental problems, sleeplessness and diminished vision as common problems. Around 20–30 per cent of them had osteoporosis. Majority of them did not visit doctor frequently. Female elderly self-caregivers faced common health problems such as diabetes, insomnia and osteoporosis. Mild and moderate degree of depression was also noticed in older elderly (30 per cent).

Knowledge assessment showed that more than 50 per cent of the elderly male self-caregivers knew about ageing but 40 per cent had poor knowledge about physiological changes and medical and health problems during ageing. Nutritional deficiencies were not much known to them. Most of them were also found to be ignorant about the dietary care and practices during ill health. They were found to be aware of importance of social care.

In case of elderly female self-caregivers, poor knowledge was observed regarding physiological changes (83 per cent) and medical problems (100 per cent). Half of them knew about water requirement but majority were unaware about requirement for social support.

There was marked increase in knowledge after NHE intervention which was imparted to 50 per cent of total elderly caregiver under study. Knowledge regarding ageing, physiological changes and medical health problems improved significantly after NHE intervention. Knowledge regarding diseases improved significantly. Change was also observed in their meal pattern practices. Knowledge regarding importance of exercise and psychological problems also showed improvement in half of total number of male caregivers. They also started believing in need for social care after NHE intervention.

In case of elderly female self-caregivers there was marked improvement in the knowledge of elderly female subjects with respect to various aspects of ageing. Considerable improvement in knowledge and practices were found in dietary aspects and meal pattern. There was significant improvement in knowledge regarding benefits of exercise and psychological problems.

These studies show that well designed approach of this kind can empower elderly living alone to improve quality of life and delay age related problems. However, these studies do indicate a need to focus on female self-caregivers for better understanding of dietary and medical aspects of caregiving.

Professional Caregiving

In Indian Society, cultural value and traditional practices emphasise on support and care of elderly by the family members themselves with honour and respects. However, recent changes in the size and structure of families have caused the rearrangement of the roles and functions of the members in the families. A combined effect of rise in aged population, rise in longevity and reduction on fertility accelerates shortage of proficient caregivers for the older persons. An ageing society has already given rise to special problems from health, family and social angle. Diseases and disabilities associated with ageing demands long term care. A shift from short term to long term care especially for elders with chronic illness has given rise to the requirement of large number of caregivers and longer duration of care services.

Health care system at various levels in our country is designed for the general population and no special provision appears for the care of elderly. Changes in the skill sets of our health care providers like nurses and ward boys is now required to respond to the special needs of the elderly. It is high time for nursing care of the elderly to be considered as a speciality where physical, emotional, spiritual needs of an elderly individual could be met in a highly dedicated manner.

Professional nurses willingly choose to play a role in the care of their patients. Elderly patients can be difficult to deal with and need special sympathetic care and support. Their special needs include nutrition, health and emotional support. Illness can effect people differently and sometimes fear, frustration and growing dependency may reflect in irritation and anger in behaviour of the elderly. This needs to be dealt with patience and loving care. Care of older patients is seen as an unpopular choice by many nurses and may lead to problems in delivering of care. There is a need for nurses to develop more positive attitudes towards the elderly patients because the importance of psycho-social care is often undervalued in the current health care set up (Cooper and Coleman, 2001). High quality caregivers are not easily available and there is a need to sensitise professional caregiving staff in Indian hospitals and home care situation. Capacity building of such caregivers who are given special professional training about care of elderly in different conditions and about specific physiological and psychological changes during old age can go a long way in achieving better management and help in speeding up the recovery process.

Considering these above facts, authors team conducted a study using action oriented approach and assess the impact of nutrition health education on the knowledge and practices of the professional caregivers of the elderly (Mehta et al., 2010).

In initial study phase, fifty elderly caregivers were given need based NHE intervention with the help of a NHE booklet and verbal counseling. The intervention was reinforced in a training workshop for improvement of hospital based care of the elderly.

Initial data before NHE intervention of 6 weeks revealed lack of knowledge amongst caregivers about various aspects regarding elderly such as the physiological changes seen in elderly and health problems commonly faced by the elderly, nutritional deficiencies affecting the elderly and the dietary services for preventing these nutritional deficiencies. There was poor knowledge about fluid requirement and care during tube feeding. Caregivers were also unaware about the psychological problems faced by the elderly persons, their causes and solutions. However, most of the caregivers treated the elderly subjects with respect, politeness and reported awareness regarding need for social support.

Post intervention data showed that there was improvement in the knowledge of caregivers regarding physiological changes in old age, medical problems faced by elderly, care in tube feeding, fluid intake and psychological problems. Marked improvement was also found in the knowledge of caregivers regarding nutritional disorders in elderly and feeling the need for geriatric ward.

Practices of ensuring adequate fluid intake by elderly patients, appropriate care and privileges for the elderly patients showed an improvement.

The overall findings of the study indicated that NHE intervention proved to be successful in bringing about improvement in the knowledge and practices of female caregivers regarding health care of elderly.

The appendix 6 may be referred for making tool for training the caregivers regarding nutrition health education of elderly.

Caring for the older is always a challenge and the older the person is, the more difficult it becomes. Burden of caregiving is enormous. A sudden heart attack, a broken hip or limb, side effects of medicines which cause allergies or respiratory and digestive infections which surface all the time may cause extra demands and may cause need to shift elderly patients under professional caregivers.

The goal of organising health services for older people should be to maintain their autonomy with due concern of their self respect and welfare of the careers. The ideal system for health care of the elderly does not exist in our society. There is growing need to create institutions which can train the caregivers for general and specific conditions of elderly and provide placements to them for needy patients. Such centers which act as home care providers can contribute great deal to elderly care in domiciliary setting.

References

Cooper S.A. and Coleman P.G. (2001), Caring for older person : An exploration of perceptions using personal construct theory, age and ageing, 30: 399-402.

Dey A.B. (2003), Health care for older people : A Manual for Trainers of Community Health Workers, Department of Medicine, All India Institute of Medical Sciences, New Delhi.

Mehta P, Chauhan K., Bhatt, T. and Kohle, P. (2010), Assessment of Knowledge and Prctices of professional caregivers (nurses) of elderly (> 75 yrs): Impact evaluation of need based NHE intervention regarding care of elderly, Journal of Indian Academy of Geriatrics, 6: 150-154.

Mehta P and Shringarpure B (2004), Role of antioxidants in health and diseases during ageing process, Unpublished doctoral dissertation, Department of Foods and Nutrition, The M.S. University, Baroda, Vadodara.

Morimoto, T., Schreineer, A.S., and A Sano H (2003). Caregiver burden and health related quality of life among Japanese stroke caregivers, Age Ageing, 32 (2): 218-223.

Panchal N, Chauhan K and Mehta P., 2005. A study on knowledge and practices of caregivers of the elderly(≥ 75 years) and impact of NHE on elderly's health, Indian Journal of Gerontology, 19 (4) : 439–46.

Prasad, D.B. and Rani, I.N. (2007), Older persons and caregiver burden and satisfaction in rural family context, Indian Journal Gerentology, Vol. 21, No. 2 pp. 216-232.

8

Some Useful Information

"Reaching the Unreached"

—By Authors

Some important information related to elderly's health are given appendices 1 to 8.

In addition, selected organisations working elderly are listed below along with detail information on National Policies for Older Persons.

A: LIST OF ORGANISATIONS WORKING FOR ELDERLY IN INDIA

Nightingales Medical Trust

337, 2nd Cross, 1st Block, R T Nagar, Bangalore - 560032
Ph: 91 80 23548444, 23548555, Fax: 91 80 23548999
Email:nhhs@bgl.vsnl.net.in
Website: http://www.nightingaleseldercare.com/index.htm

The Longevity Centre (TLC),India

CASP Bhavan, 132/2, Plot # 3,Pashan-Baner Link Road, Pune 411 021
Tel : 91 (20) 25862844-46/49
Fax : 91 (20) 25862836 & 25862849
Email : longevitic@vsnl.net
Website: http://www.ilcindia.org/

(ARDSI) Alzheimer's & Related Disorders Society of India

Head Office: Guruvayur Road, P.B. No. 53 Kunnamkulam - 680 503, Kerala
Email: alzheimr@md2.vsnl.net.in
Mumbai office: BMC School Bldg (II/room 127), JJ Hospital Complex,
Byculla, Mumbai-400008.
Tel: 91+022+ 23742479
Email: people4sc@gmail.com
Website : http://www.mykerala.net/alzheimer/ardsi_man_01.html

The Family Welfare Agency

Near B D D Chawl NO: 10, N M Joshi Marg, Lower Parel (E), Mumbai - 13
Ms Swati Ingole at 91-022-24015150;
Email: tfwas@yahoo.co.in

Society for Serving Seniors (SSS)

30, Gruhalakshmi Colony,
Secunderabad-500015,
Andhra Pradesh
Phone : 27846631
Email:vyasamoorthy@gmail.com
Website: http://societyforservingseniors.satyamcsr.org/

Harmony

Maker Chambers IV, Fourth Floor, 222, Nariman Point, Mumbai, Maharashtra-400021.
Office: 2-278-5400
Fax: 2-285-2217
Website: http://www.harmonyindia.org/hportal/home.jsp

Helpage India

C-14 Qutab Institutional Area, New Delhi–110016
Ph: 011 41688955-56
E-mail: headoffice@helpageindia.org
Website: http://www.harmonyindia.org/hportal/home.jsp

Dignity Foundation

BMC School Building, Topiwala Lane, Opp. Lamington Road Police Station, Mumbai-400 007.
Telephone: 23898079/23841845/23814356 Fax: 23898082
Email: dignity@vsnl.com
Website: http://www.dignityfoundation.com/index.php

B: NATIONAL POLICY FOR OLDER PERSONS (1999)

Courtesy : Dr. D V Bala

Demographic ageing is the global phenomenon that has hit Indian structure also. Life expectancy at birth has shown a steady rise from 24 years in 1901 to 42 years in 1961 and to 67 years in 2011. Elderly population is one of the most vulnerable groups and needs special attention. The National policy for Older Persons (1999) is the outcome of this need. It seeks to assure older persons that their concerns are national concerns and they will not live unprotected, ignored or marginalised.

Goal: Goal of the policy is the well-being of older persons. It aims to strengthen their legitimate place in society and help older persons to live their life with purpose, dignity and peace.

Objectives

1. To encourage individuals to make various provisions such as health and social insurance for their own as well as their spouse's old age;
2. To encourage families to take care of their older family members;
3. To enable and support voluntary and nongovernmental organizations to supplement the care provided by the family, with great emphasis on non institutional care;
4. To provide care and protection to the vulnerable elderly especially widows, frail, handicapped, abused and destitute elderly;
5. To provide health care facilities specially suited to elderly;
6. To promote research and training facilities to train geriatric caregivers and organisers of services for the elderly;

7. To continuously evaluate and upgrade existing services and programs for older people me.
8. To facilitate and strengthen inter sectoral partnerships in the field; and
9. To create awareness regarding elder persons to develop themselves into fully independent citizens.

Implementation Strategy

A. Preparation of plan of action for operationalization of the National Policy;

B. Setting up of separate Bureau for older persons in Ministry of Social Justice and Empowerment;

C. Setting up of Directorates of older persons in the states;

D. Three Yearly Public Review of implementation of policy;

E. Setting up of a National Council for Older Persons headed by Minister for Social Justice & Empowerment (Representatives from Central Ministries, States, Non-Official members representing NGOs, academic bodies, media and experts);

F. Establishment of Autonomous National Association of Older Persons; and

G. Encouraging the participation of legal self government. Steps Already Taken for Implementation of NPOP Setting up of Council.

A national Council for Older persons (NCOP) under the chairpersonship of the Minister of State for Social Justice & Empowerment has been set up consisting 39 members. The NCOP is the designated office for receiving suggestions, complaints and grievances from older persons. A seven member working group has also been constituted from amongst the members of NCOP.

Aadhar

The Ministry has also commissioned "Aadhar", as a secretariat of the NPOP in 1999. It is being coordinated by

"Agewell Foundation". Aadhar is an initiative in the direction of empowering the elderly population of India to find satisfactory solutions to the problems as per their felt needs through coordination of voluntary efforts and administrative initiatives. Aadhar is attending to requests for intervention received from all over the country. In addition to the regular activities, a process of identification has been initiated by Aadhar for setting up voluntary action groups in all 578 districts of the country for better implementation of ideas and to provide for older persons effectively at the local level. The plan of action 2000–2005 operationalisers the NPOP to take up various initiatives.

OLD Age Social and Income Security (OASIS) Project

An eight-member expert committee was nominated to examine policy questions connected with old age and to make concrete recommendations for actions so that every young worker can built up enough savings during his/her working life, which would serve as a shield against poverty in their old age and reduce the burden on the state. The social Defense Bureau is taking the necessary actions for the implementation of the recommendations of the report.

Reference

J Kishore (2011), National Health Programmes, 9th edition, Century Publications.

9

Remarks and Recommendations

"Add life to years and not years to life"

–Unknown

Based on the chapters in the book

1. Almost all Indian studies report inadequate nutrient intake and compromised meal pattern in geriatric population. Scenario is worst in poor economic section and elderly living alone.
2. Oral cavity problems and respiratory problems rank highest amongst health problems of elderly.
3. Minor health complaints decrease with improvement in nutritional status.
4. Mental performance also improves with improvement in nutritional status
5. Essence of studies on older elderly centenarians is simple lifestyle, regularity, stress free life and adequate food intake, social interactions and engagement in activities requiring physical and mental efforts.
6. For institutions like day care for aged or old age homes, following may be considered:
    a. All institutions should include recreational activities, lift, telephone and banking facilities.

b. Facilities for transport (within the campus for those not able to walk and for emergencies) and attendants for special needs and call for help during emergency should be made available.

c. Inclusion of vegetable especially green leafy vegetables and fruits should be compulsory in the diet.

d. Soups and juices, khakhras and handy food should be made available easily (paid or free).

e. Donors need to be educated not to donate sweets and fried foods on occasions. Donation of healthy food items and hygienically safe items may be encouraged.

f. Pleasant atmosphere may be provided with joyful activities for attainment of satisfaction, mental alertness and pleasure.

7. Depressed elderly may be dealt separately for their emotional and social needs. Treatment measures and good diet should be started as early as possible to improve mental status.

8. Community survey can be undertaken to detect mental health disorders and patients may be provided with suitable healthcare.

9. High fibre, low bulk, low fat food should be recommended for elderly along with ample fluids.

10. White poison like sweet, sugar, salt, ghee, butter, oil, may be restricted.

11. Easy to chew and swallow and easily digestible food may be given in quantity frequently.

12. Food technologies like ARF and fermentation may be tried for elderly with swallowing disorders.

13. Oral cavity problems should be attended immediately and regular body checkups may be done.

14. Helpline of 24-hrs for getting quality help such as attendees, nurses and doctors, medicines, blood etc.

15. Special benefits may be made available at public places like bus-stands and rickshaw-stands, or common benches in malls or elsewhere.
16. Private and public hospital Practitioners, clinics etc. should give priority to elderly patients without much waiting. concession in fees may also be given
17. Special geriatric hospitals and wards should be established.
18. Education regarding geriatric care may be made compulsory at all levels of education programmes.

Appendices

Appendix-1

"Health And Nutrition Care For Elderly"
(Training Module for Healthcare of Elderly)

Developed by: Prof Pallavi Mehta (Retd. Head)
Dr Komal Chauhan (Associate Professor)
Department of Foods and Nutrition
Faculty of Family and Community Sciences
The M.S. University of Baroda, Vadodara

Ageing is not a disease,

But it is a biological process.

During ageing the capacity of working cell decreases.

The population of aged is increasing globally, physical capacity declines and

become dependent economically.

For successful ageing, nutritious food plays a very important role.

Along with physical and mental changes in the body, their likes, nutrition needs and amount of food also changes. This directly affects health and nutritional status. Therefore with ageing, improvement in quality of life is very important.

To attain this at right time it is required to build self confidence in elderly that will help to sustain against physical, mental, social and emotional changes in life.

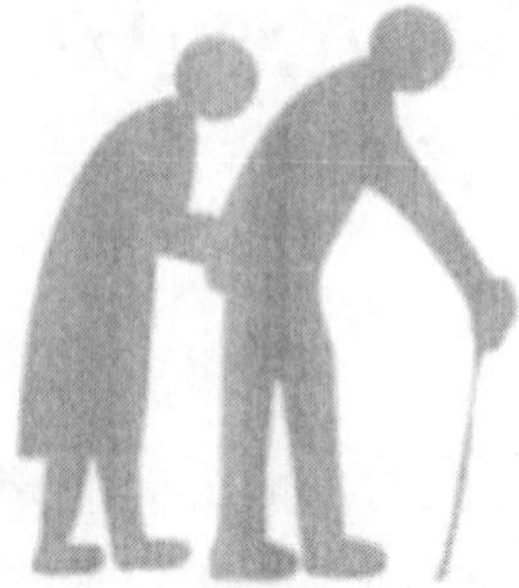

Danger Signs during Ageing

- Malnutrition (under or over nutrition)
- Physical dependency
- Side effects of medicines
- Accidents and falls
- Problem of sound sleep
- Oral cavity problems
- Non communicable diseases like diabetes, heart disease and cancer

- Constipation
- Anemia
- Problems of hearing and vision
- Locomotor problems: Arthritis, Fractures, paralysis etc.
- Mental tension, memory loss, depression, shock, isolation
- Prostrate problems, etc.

Care during Eating

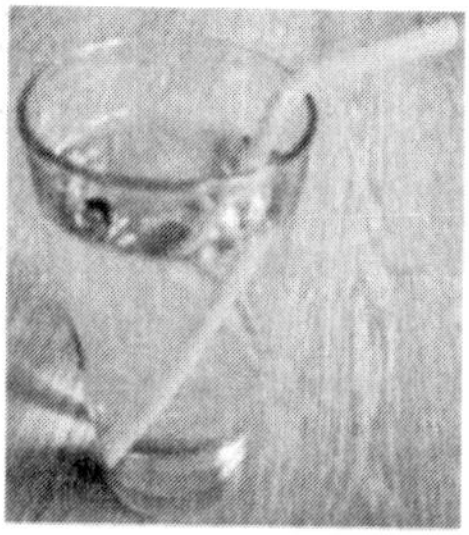

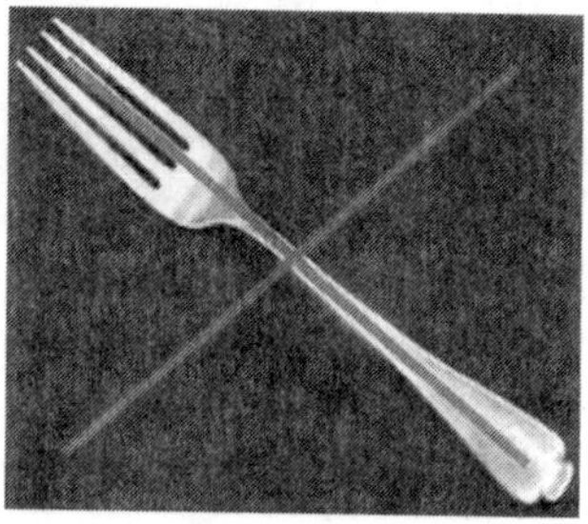

- Prefer straw for liquid foods
- Do not use fork for eating

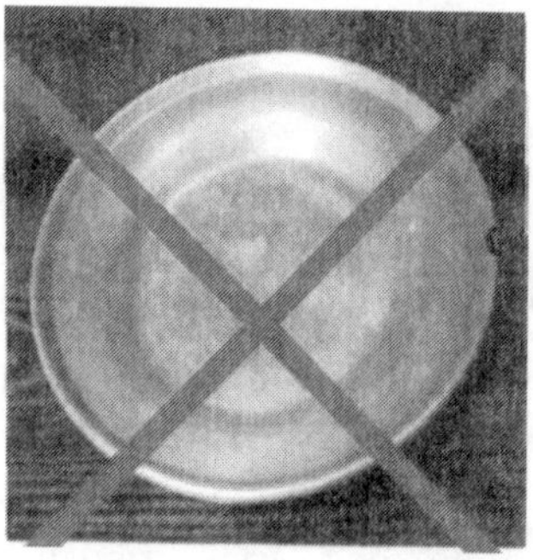

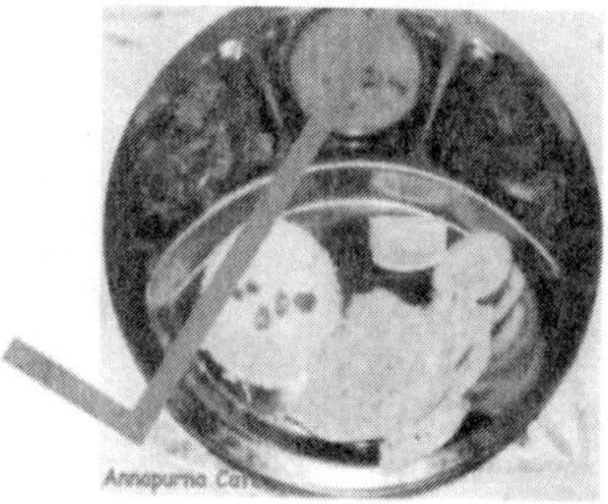

- Use plates with compartments for comfortable eating

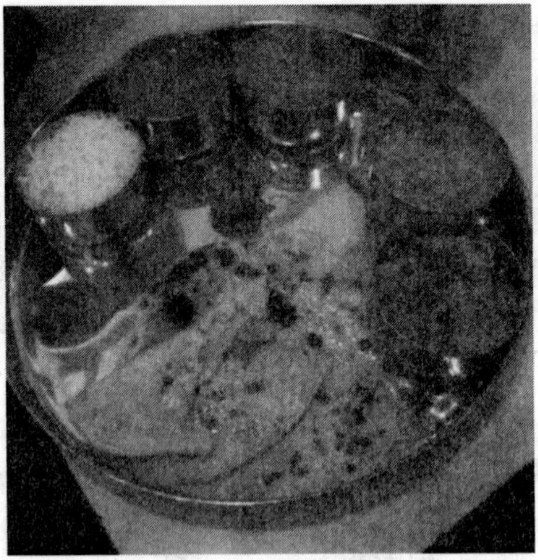

- Place the foods in plate clockwise manner so that it can be explained to elderly with dim vision

SLEEPING

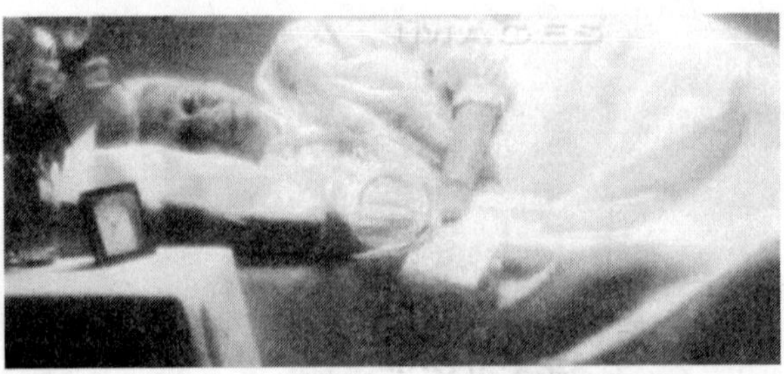

- Wake up and bed timings should be regular, it helps in maintaining good health.
- Room of the elderly should be airy, spacious and comfortable. Before going to bed drink a glass of warm milk for sound sleep

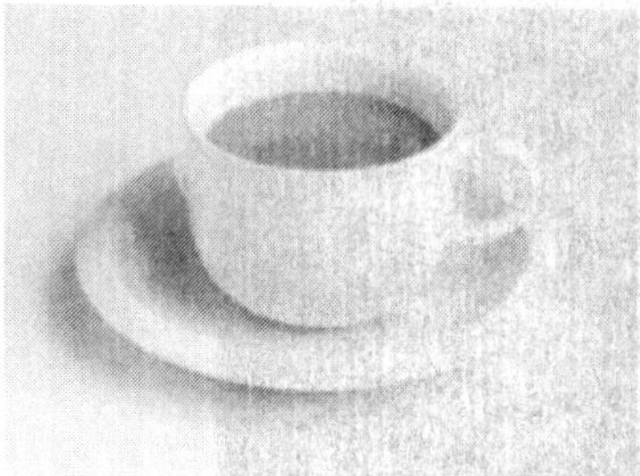

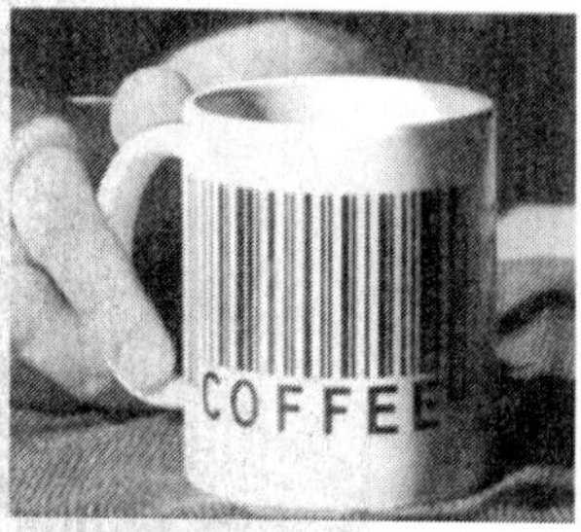

- Do not drink tea/coffee in the evening/night

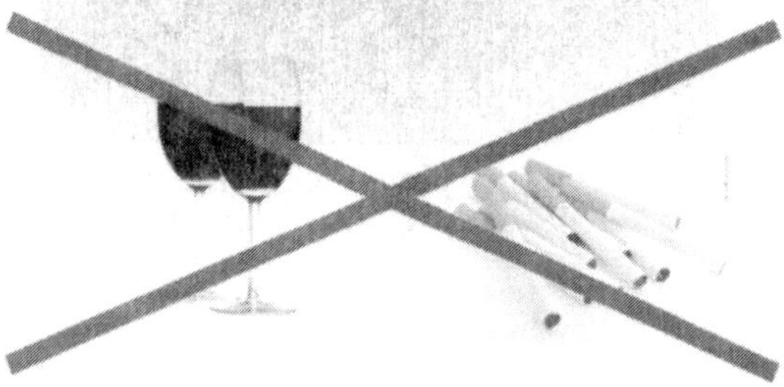

- Avoid cigarette or Hard drink

Oral Cavity Problem

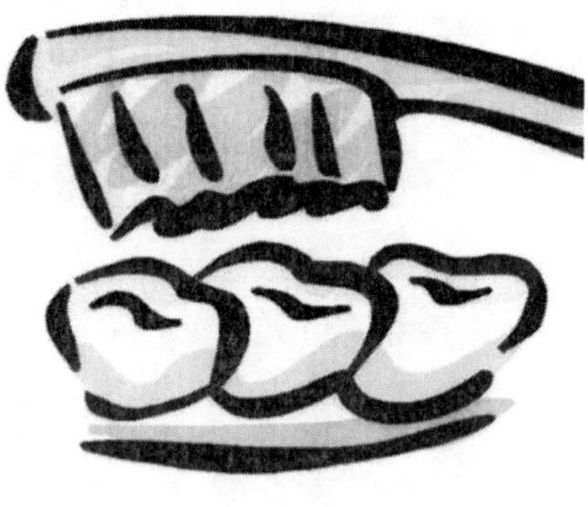

- Brush regularly with care
- Elderly often face problem of dryness in mouth, therefore make them drink water frequently and keep a source of drinking water nearby.

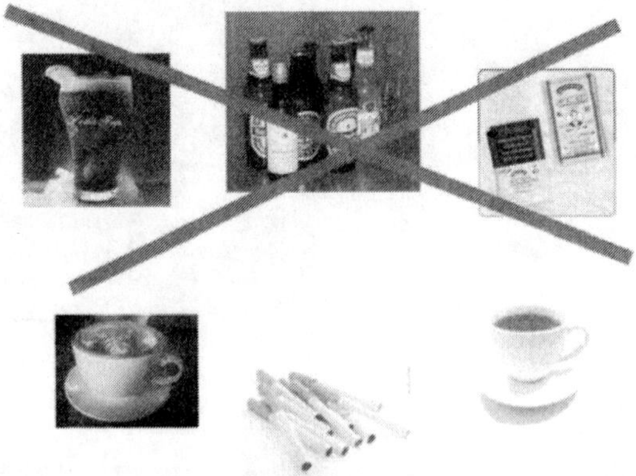

- Elderly with partial teeth, without teeth should be given food which is easy to chew and swallow like Soft, semi-solid or liquid e.g. Soup, porridge, khichadi, boiled veg and fruits.

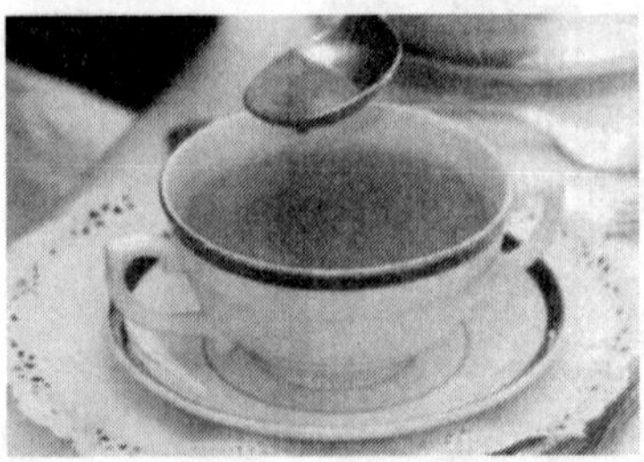

Care of Oral Cavity

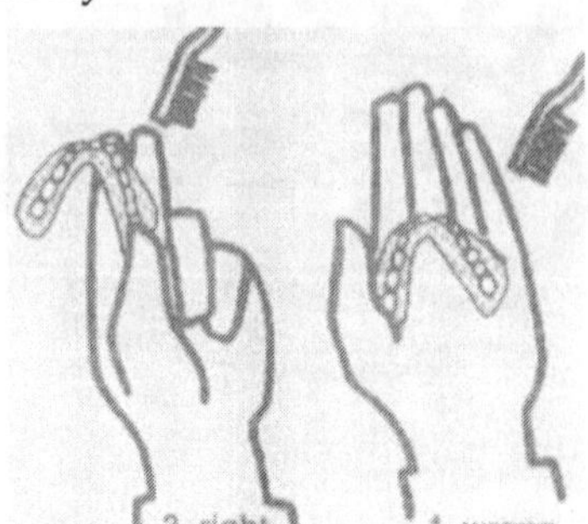

- For people using artificial dentures

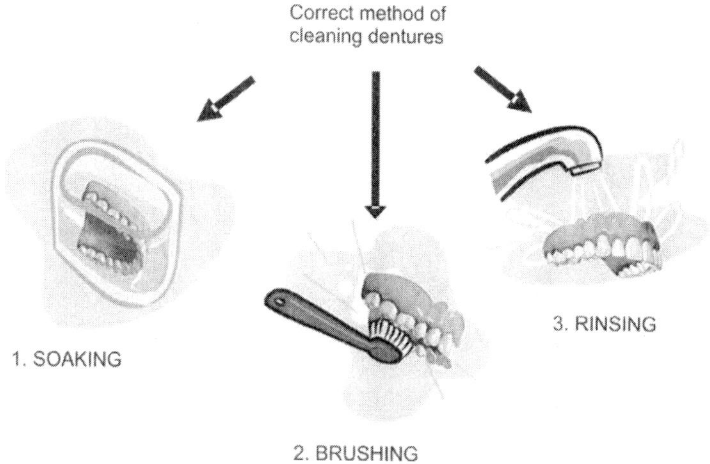

Care for Diabetics

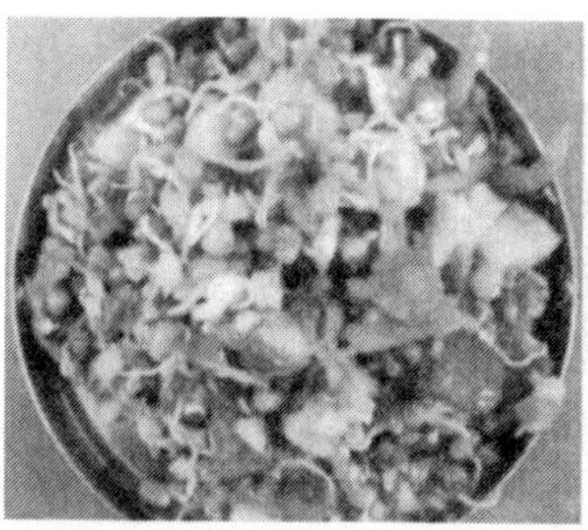

Take balanced food

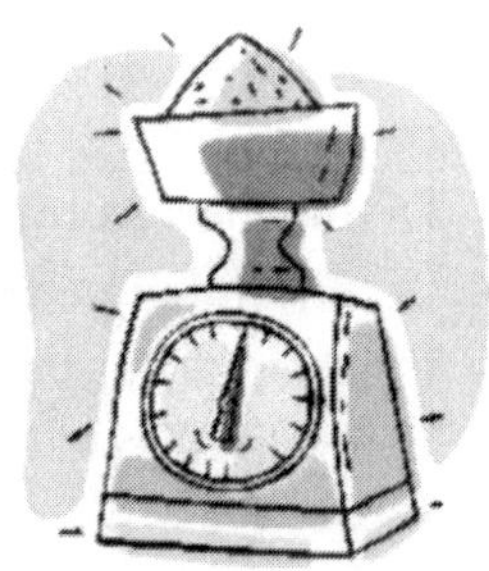

Take required quantity food only

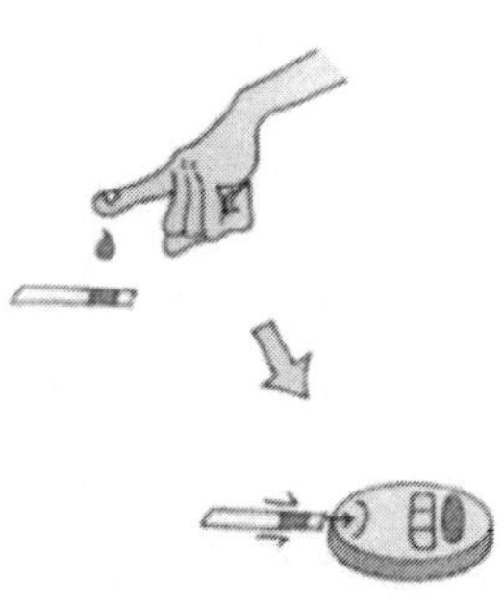

Check regular blood glucose levels

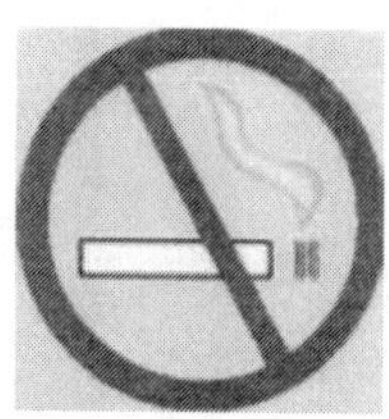

Avoid smoking

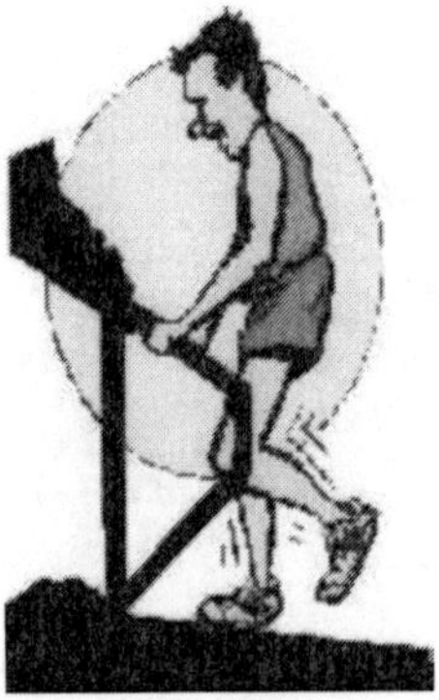

Exercise regularly

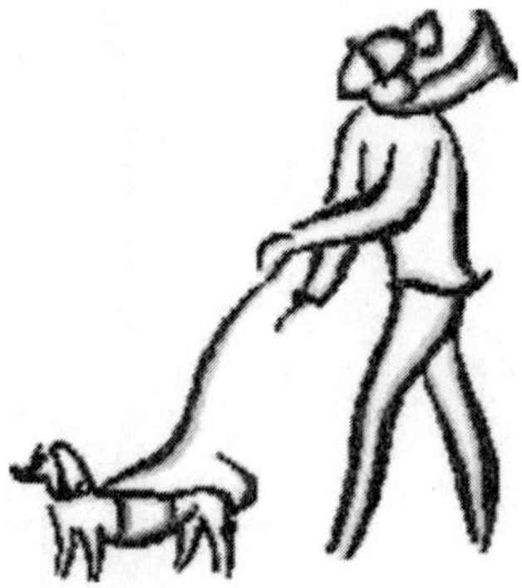

Walk for minimum 30 min daily

Avoid following foods in diabetes.

- Fried foods: Puri, samosa, pakodas, farshan, etc.
- Sweets, sugar, jaggery, cakes, chocolates, confectionaries
- Dry fruits: groundnuts, almond, raisins, dates, etc.
- Cold drinks (carbonated), canned juices, alcohol.
- Fruits: grapes, banana, ripe mango, chiku, litchi,
- Vegetables: potato, sweet potato, tapioca, tubers.
- Whole milk, cream, butter, ghee, egg yolk, meat.

Why

- Because they are foods with High Glycaemic Index.
- All carbohydrate foods are absorbed faster and raise blood glucose levels differently in body. Foods like sugar, jiggery, potato raise blood glucose levels very fast so they are called as high glycemic index foods.

Therefore

- Patients with diabetes should consume very less amount of foods with high glycaemic index

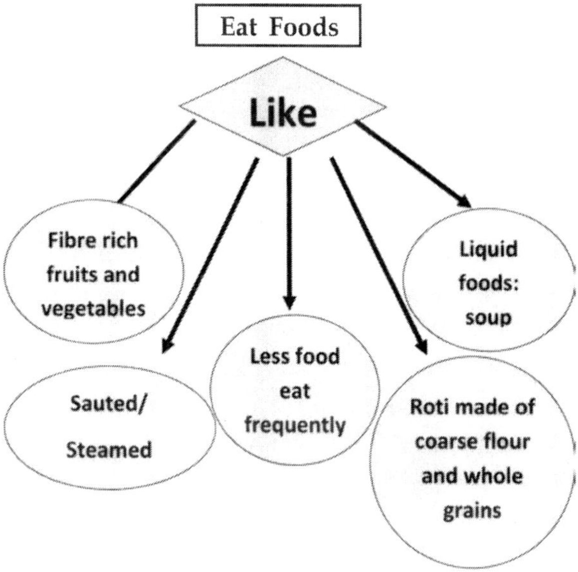

Care for conditions of High blood pressure/heart disease

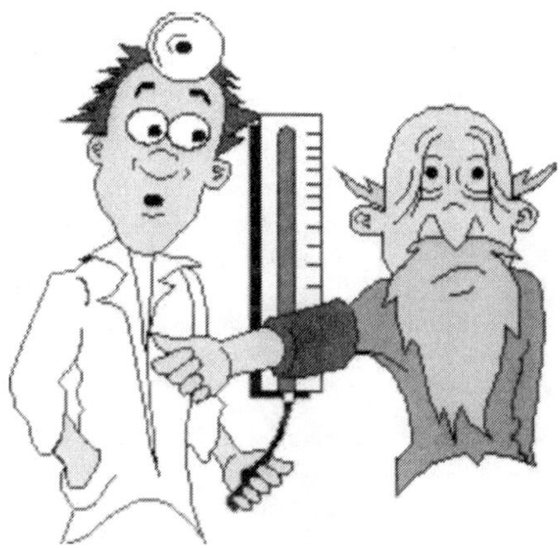

- Do not feast, do not fast.
- Include more amount of vegetables and fruits in diet.
- Prefer whole fresh fruits sugar free juice.
- Consume chopped/grated raw salad (salt free) daily.
- Use mixture or blend of oils instead saturated fats like ghee, butter, coconut oil, etc.

- Do not consume extra fried foods, baked foods using hydrogenated fats like dalda.
- Prefer skimmed milk (low fat) only.
- Decrease use of salt in foods.
- Prefer vegetarian foods more.
- Non veg. foods like meat should be boiled before cooking and discard water to reduce salt content in it.
- Minimise use of baking soda or sodium bicarbonate.

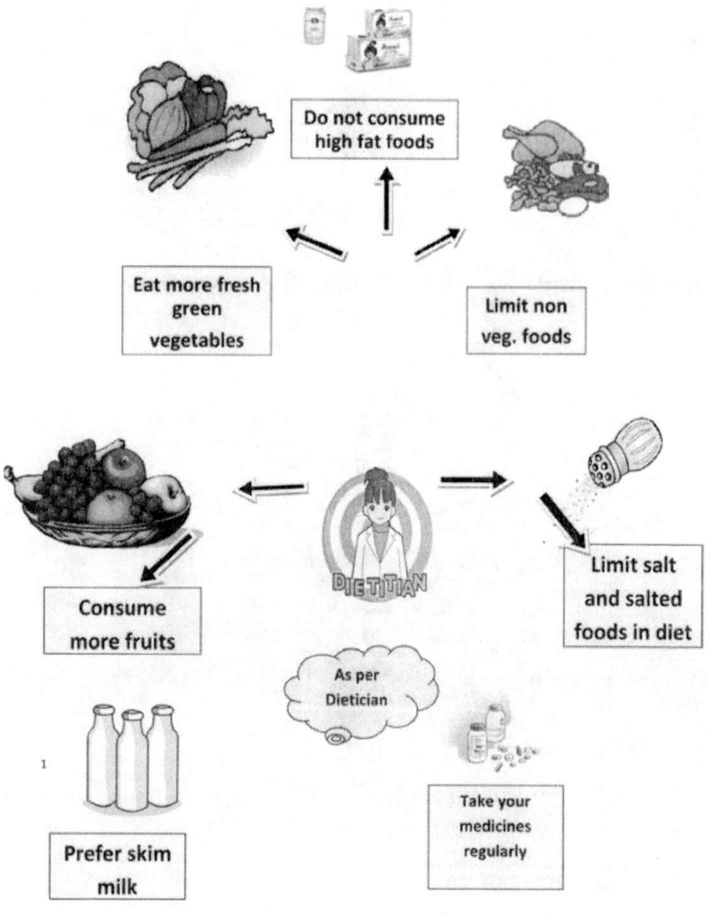

Constipation

Elderly has common complaint of constipation. Cause could be foods, lack of fluids and exercise and side effects of medicines.

- Consume whole grains, green leafy vegetables, whole fruits daily.

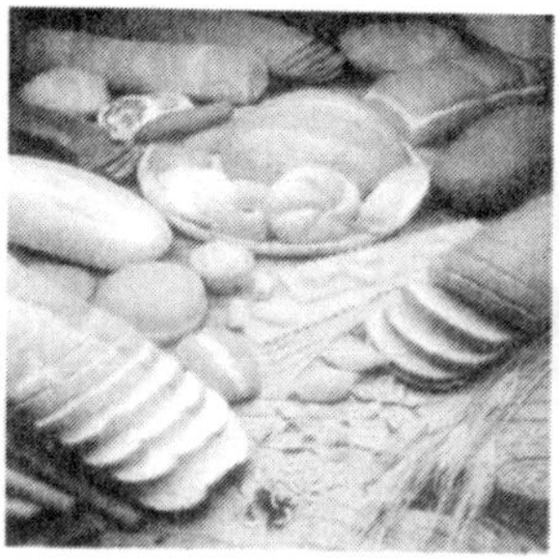
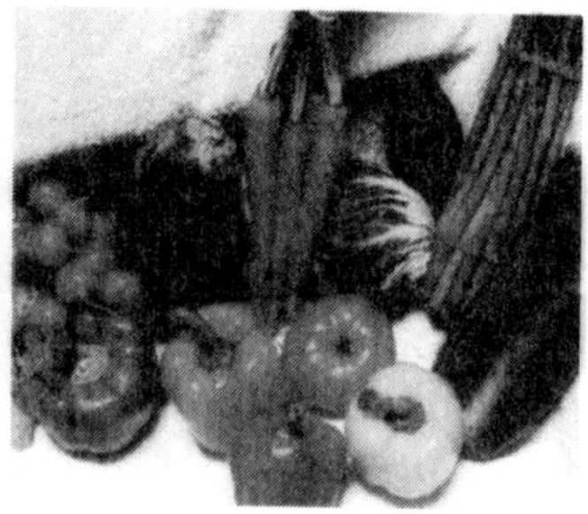

- If liquid is not restricted than minimum 8 glass of water be consumed (1.5 - 2 L).
- Keep water source near the bed of elderly so that they can use it frequently.
- Consumption of coffee, outside foods, antacid or over use of laxatives can lead to constipation

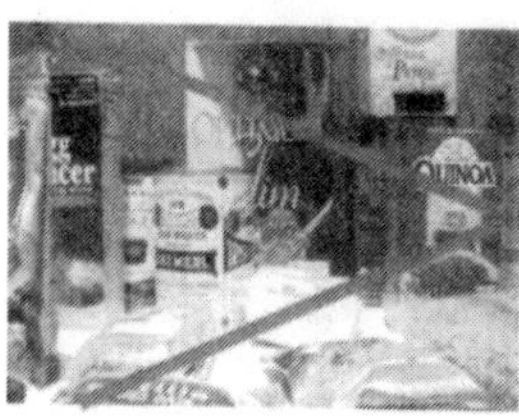
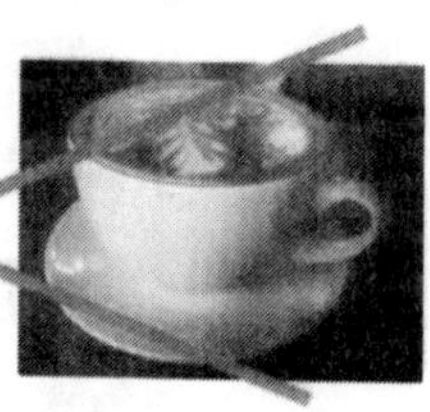

- Patient should do light exercise like yoga, walking, etc. to relieve from constipation.

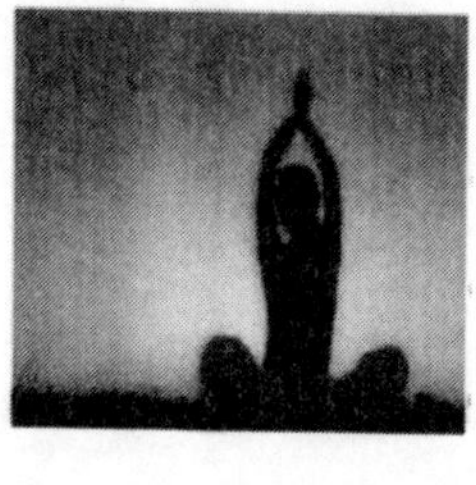

Acidity

- Remaining hungry for long can lead to acidity. Other causes are outside foods, spicy foods, high fried food consumption, smoking, addiction to alcohol, etc. so avoid them.

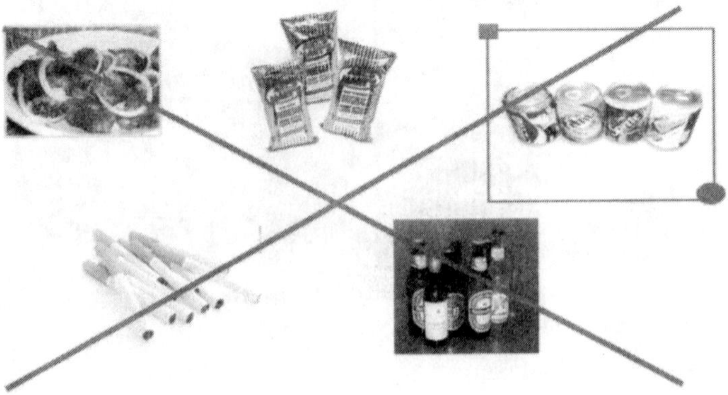

- Drinking cold milk helps to reduce acidity.

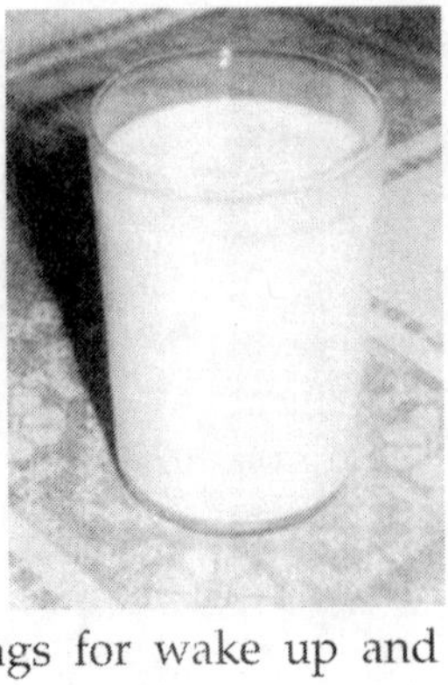

- Regular timings for wake up and bed also helps to prevent it.

Hearing

- With ageing hearing impairment takes place.

- Try to use sign language for communication with them.

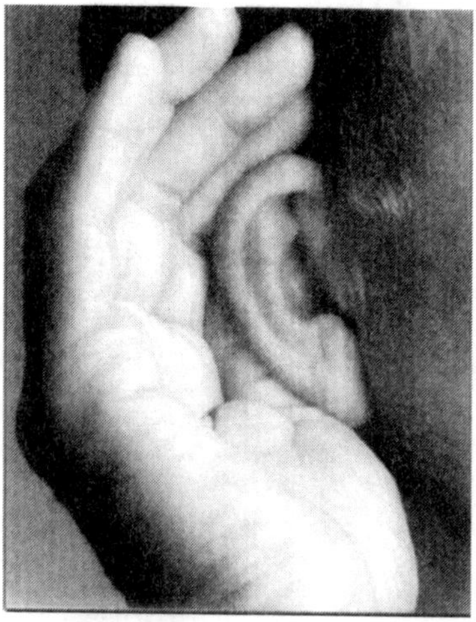

- Explain them about disorder and benefits of taking medicines patiently.
- Try to convince elderly for benefits of hearing aid and explain how to use with utmost care.

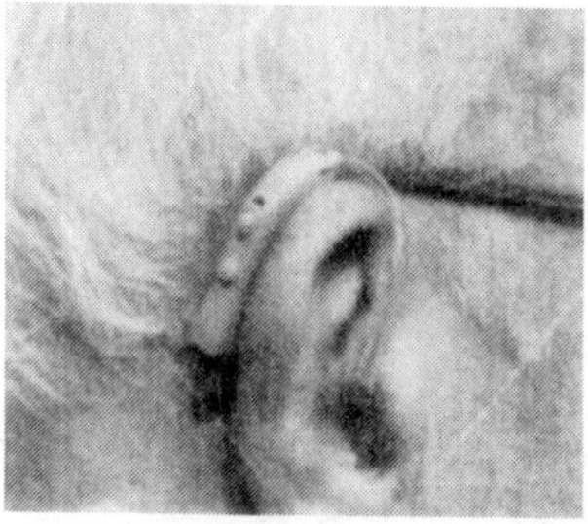

Poor Eye Sight

- On ageing, vision impairment is also seen.
- Help them in routine task like getting up, eating, walking, etc.
- Keep their spectacles handy.
- Proper lighting and use of walking stick, walker, wheel chair be encouraged.

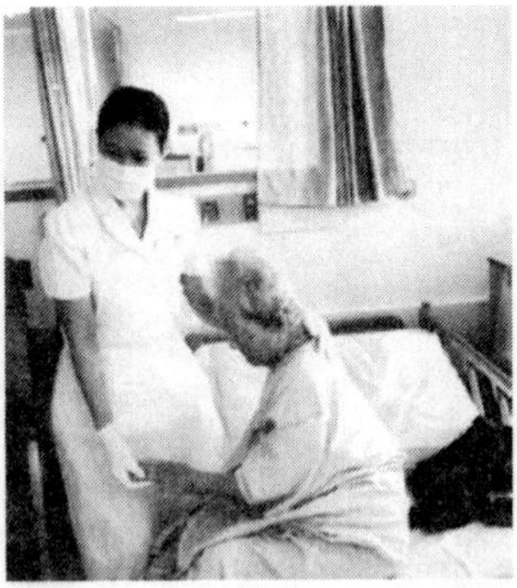

Cancer

- Patient should be due to the disease given balanced appetite decrease diet, which is very and requirement important. Of nutritious food increases.

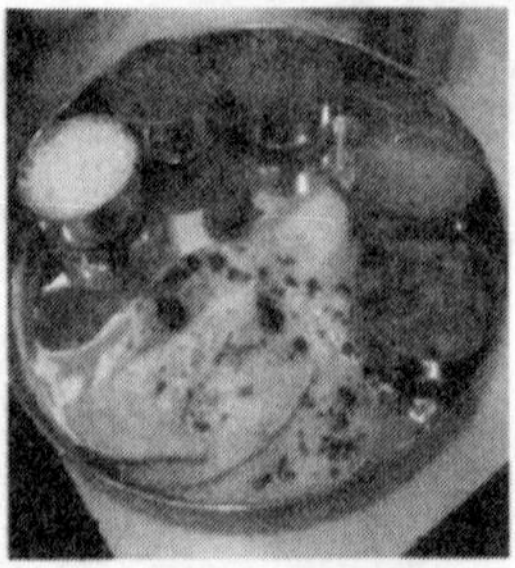

- Therefore it becomes very important to care for their food.

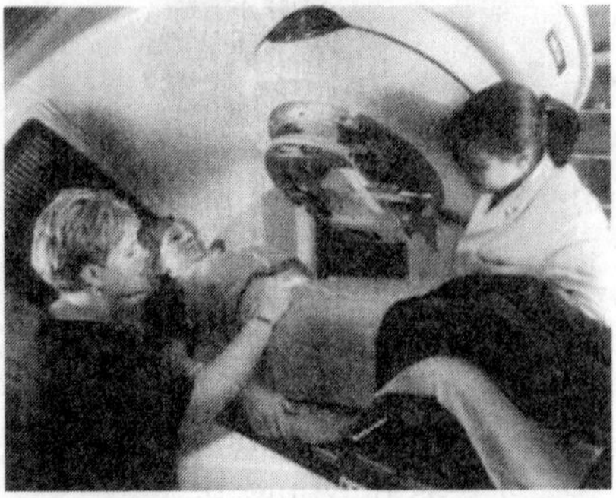

- Explain patient about the medical treatment procedure.

- Let patient be relaxed and tension free for proper treatment and its outcome.
- Prepare patient for chemotherapy and radiation. Council them and make them tension free.

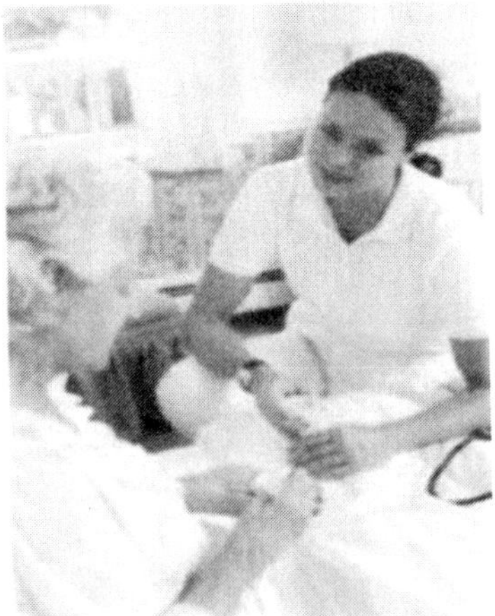

- Family members should be briefed about the disease and its care.

Locomotor Problem

- Elderly people should be helped in moving with care that they would not slip or fall.

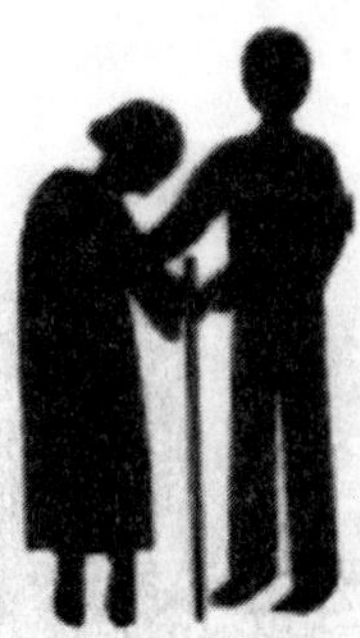

- Floor mats and carpets should be avoided in the room of the elderly as it would be a hindrance, causing falls and fracture.

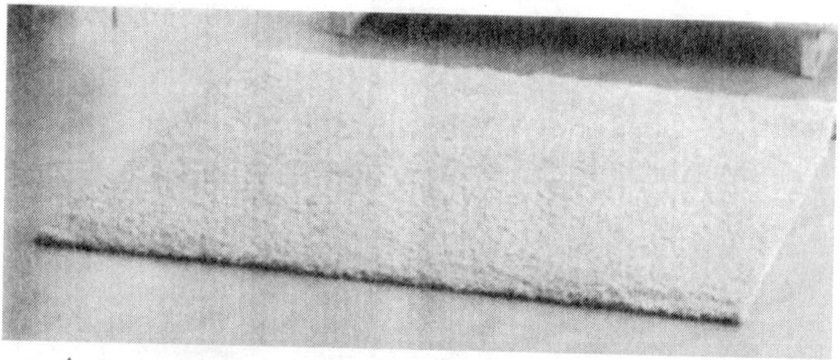

- Areas near staircase and corridors should be well lighted.

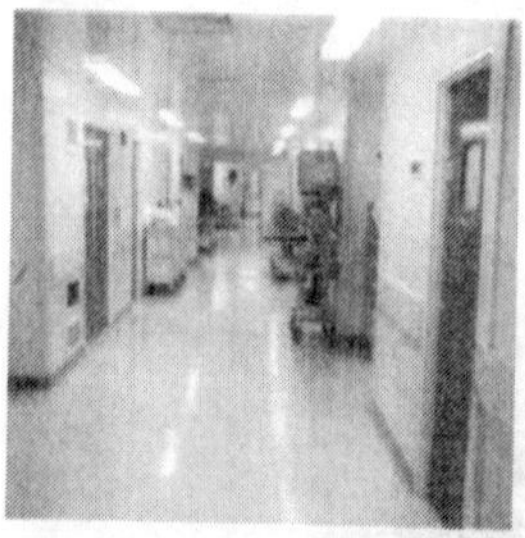

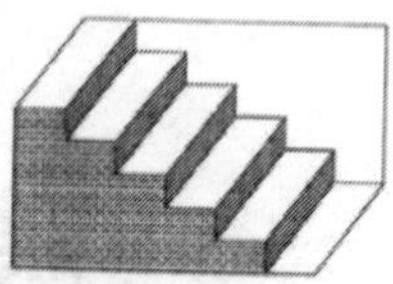

- Elderly should always prefer flat foot wears as they are comfortable to wear and walk.

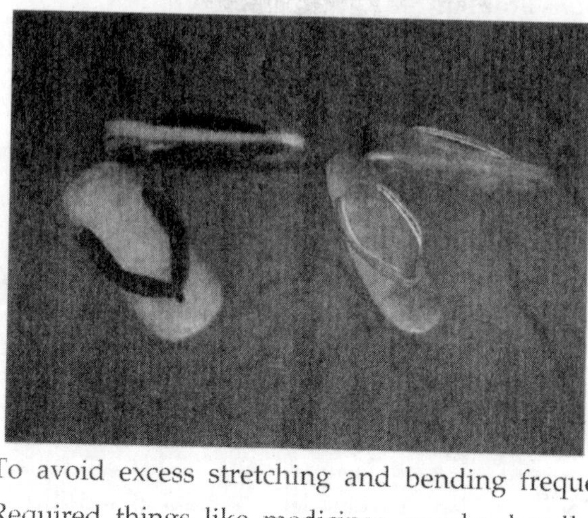

- To avoid excess stretching and bending frequently.
- Required things like medicines, specks, handkerchief, etc. should be kept on table in nearby places.

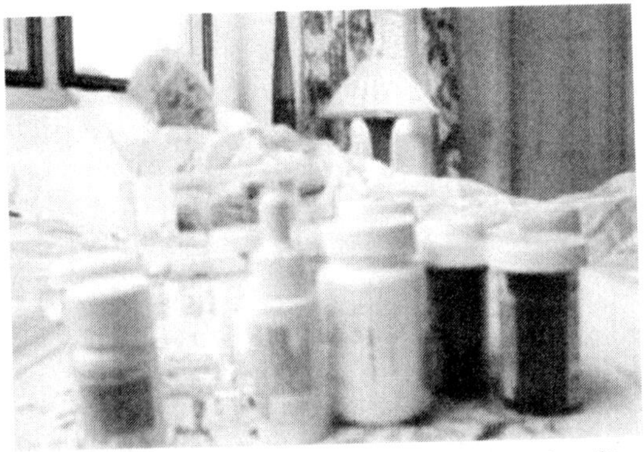

- If elderly is suffering from Parkinson's disease help him to carry out routine activities.

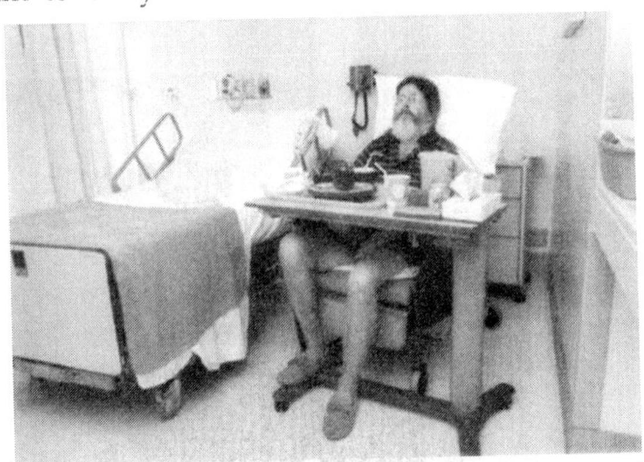

- If patient has problem of excess salivation, clean his mouth frequently to maintain his personnel hygiene.

How to Help Elderly with Locomotor Problem?

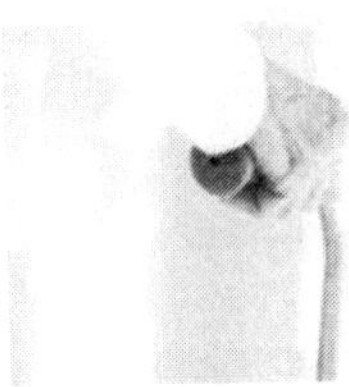

Help him to use walking stick

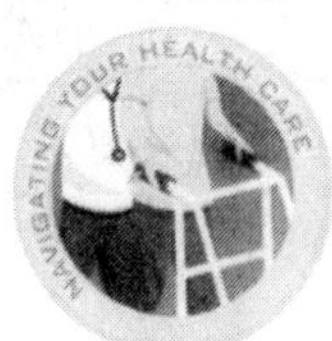

Use of proper aid like walker to avoid falls

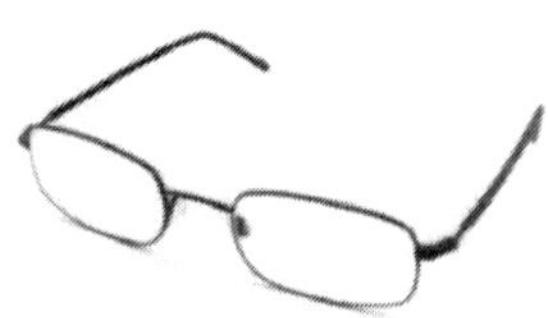

With use of correct number specks

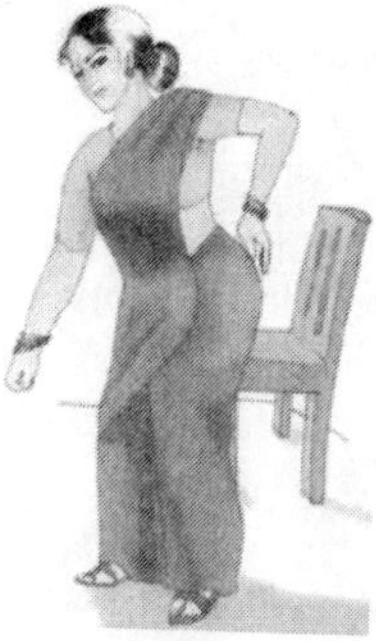

To remove hindrance in between

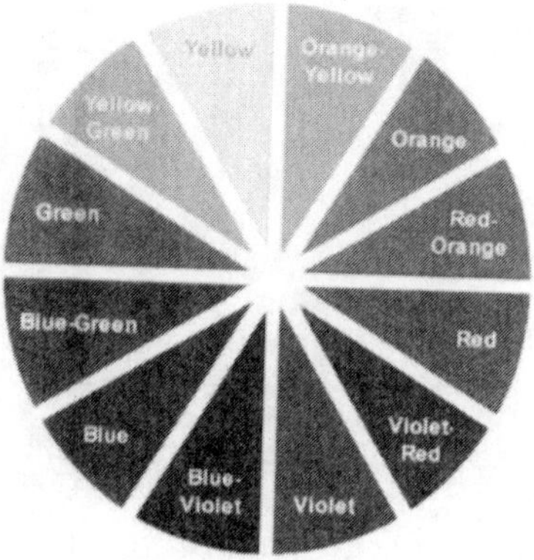

Help to use colour chart

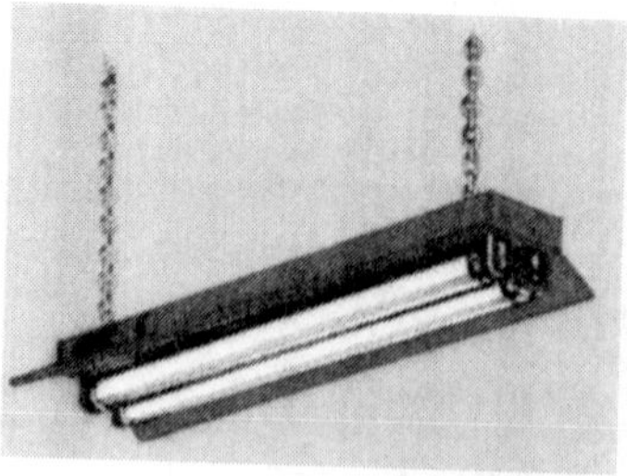

Proper light facilities

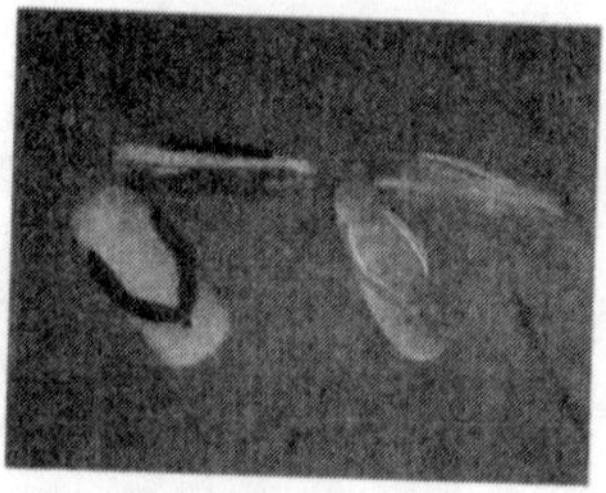

Making use of comfortable foot wears

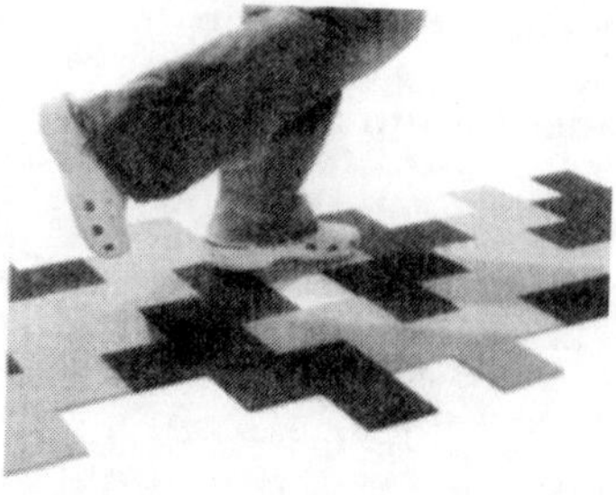

Flooring should be non slippery (anti skid)

MEDICATION

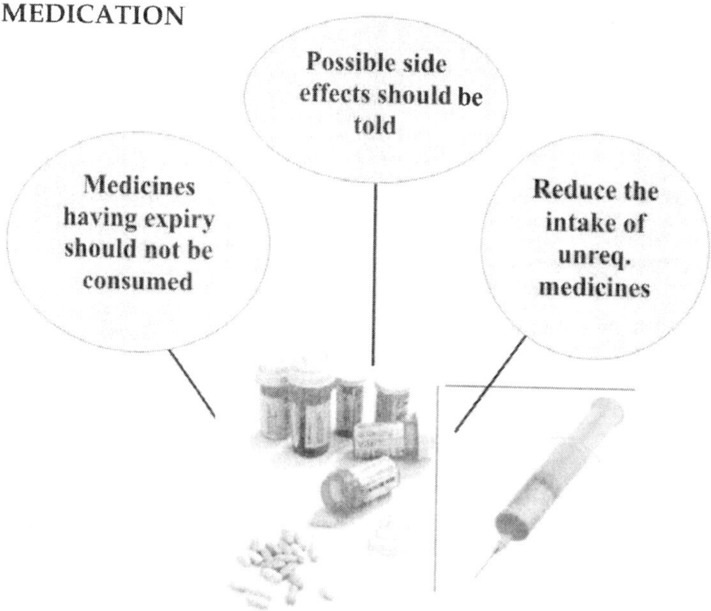
Possible side effects should be told
Medicines having expiry should not be consumed
Reduce the intake of unreq. medicines

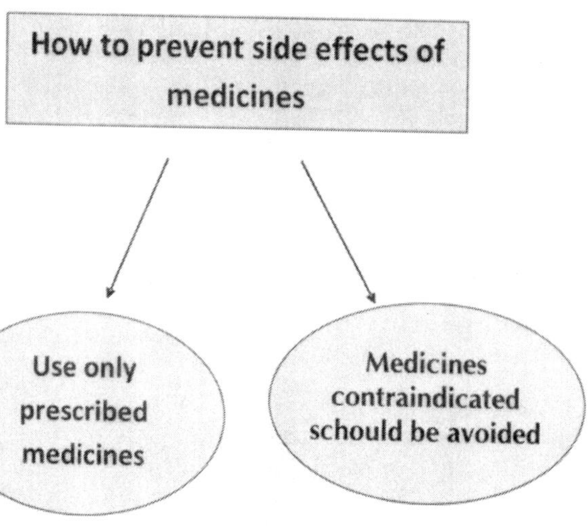
How to prevent side effects of medicines
Use only prescribed medicines
Medicines contraindicated schould be avoided

APPENDIX 2

Food Pyramid

BALANCED DIET CHART FOR ELDERLY

After advice from a dietictian one should make use of this chart for taking balanced diet

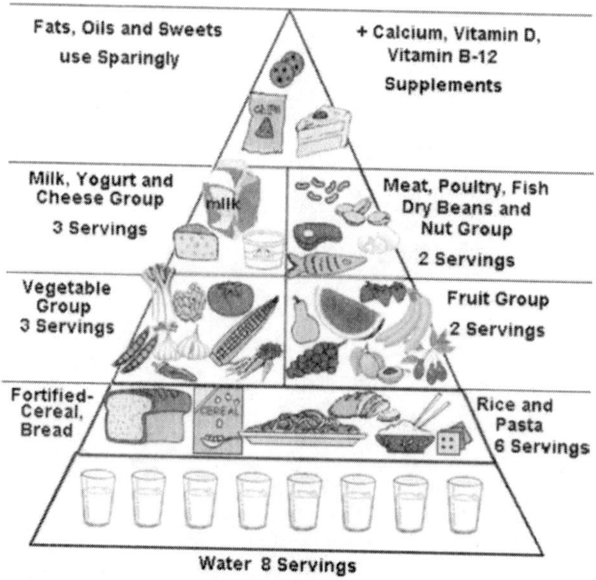

If liquid is not restricted then minimum 8 glass of drinking water is advisable (1.5 - 2 L)

APPENDIX - 3

Recommended Daily Allowance of Chief Nutrients for Elderly (Appoximate)

Sr.No.	*Nutrients*	*Daily Allowance*	
		Men	*Women*
1.	Total Calorie (kcal)	1800-2000	1600-1800
2.	Carbohydrate (g)	250-270	200-250
3.	Proteins (g)	60	50
4.	Fat (g)	20	20
5.	Iron (mg)	30	30
6.	Calcium (mg)	500	800
7.	Selenium (mg)	50	50
8.	Zinc (mg)	10	10
9.	Thiamine (mg)	1.5	1.5
10.	Riboflavin (mg)	1.5	1.5
10.	Niacin (mg)	16	16
11.	Folic Acid (Mcg)	200	180
12.	Vit E (mg)	10	10
13.	Vit C (mg)	50	50
14.	Vit B_{12} (mcg)	15	15
15.	β – carotene (μg)	2400	2400
16.	Zinc (mg)	10	10

Source: Ramamurti P V, 2008, A Book on *The Joy of Ageing Centre for Research on Ageing, Department of Psychology*, S V University, Tirupati.

Food Exchange List

Sr. no.	*Exchange*	*Approx. amount of raw foods*	*Approx. measure of raw foods*	*Energy (Kcal)*	*Protein (gm)*	*Carbohy-drate (gm)*	*Fat (gm)*
1.	Milk	250	1 cup	170	8	12	10
2 (a).	Meat	40	2 pieces or 1 egg	70	7	Neg.	5
2 (b).	Pulse	30	3 tbsp	100	7	17	Neg.
3 (a).	Vegetable A	100	½ cup	Neg.	Neg.	Neg.	Neg.
3 (b).	Vegetable B	100-150	½ cup	40	2	7	Neg.
4.	Fruits	80-100	1 portion	40	Neg.	10	Neg.
5.	Cereals	20	3 tbsp	70	2	15	Neg.
6.	Fat	5	1 tsp	45	-	-	5

APPENDIX - 4

Tips for Healty Living

- Take balanced diet.
- Do yoga meditation and exercise to remain fit.
- Regular medical check-up is must.
- Involve oneself in social activities.
- Reading and religious activity helps in preventing tension and isolation.
- Be positive.
- Maintain cleanliness.
- Avoid addictions.

Dietary Awareness

- Eat little quantity frequently.
- Eat light food in dinner.
- Prefer to drink warm milk before going to bed.
- Eat whole cereals and pulses everyday.
- Eat calcium rich food daily.
- Eat 300-500 gm of fruits and vegetables.
- Avoid tea/coffee beverages at night.
- Reduce consumption of salt, sugar and fats.
- Take regular meals daily.

- Avoid feasts and fasts.
- Avoid fast foods, processed and canned foods.

DO'S

- Eat less more frequently.
- Eat light food in the evening.
- Prefer boiled, steamed, soft and easily digestible foods.
- Include salads in the diet.
- Include calcium rich foods in the daily diet.
- Use whole grains, fruits and vegetables liberally.
- Drink one glass of warm milk before going to bed at night.
- Have two hours gap between dinner and bed time.
- Non-veg people should prefer fish and chiken instead of meat and mutton.
- Eat seasonal and local f and v abundantly.
- Give attractive foods, include likes and dislikes.

DON'T'S

- Do not skip any meal.
- Do not fast and feast.
- Ghee, sugar and salt are poisonous.
- Do not eat high fat rich non-veg food in more amounts.
- Eat spicy, fried, savoury and sweets in fewer amounts.
- Fast foods and canned foods are injurious to heart.

APPENDIX - 5

List of Old Age Homes in Gujarat

Sr. No.	Names	Contact no.
	AHMEDABAD	
1.	Jivan Sandhya Old Age Home Vanprastha Sewa Samaj, Nr. Ankur, Naranpura, Nr. Kalpataru Society	079-7475521
2.	Shah Maganlal & Keshavlal Trikamlal Trust, Nr. Income Tax Office, Ashram Road	079-546563
3.	Shree Kritincharya Pujya Shree Vijay Shankar Maharaj Bhagwat Vidyapith Vanprasthashram Sola-Sarkhej, Gandhinagar Road	079-6820575
4.	Manibe Tribhovandas Old Age Home Vikasgruh, Anandnagar, Sarkhej Road, Nr. Chandranagar Bus Stand, Paldi	079-6603928
5.	Shree Manilal Gandhi Vanprasthashram Ne Cadila Crossing, Jasoda Chowkdi, Vatwa	079-5892083
6.	Shree Bharati Bapu Ashram Old Age Home, Nr. Sarkhej Railway Station	079-6820575
7.	Shree Mumbadevi Old Age Home Bhagwat Vidyapith Compound, Sola-Gandhinagar Highway	079-7484412
8.	Vatwa Jain Ashram Mah virnagar, Railway crossing, Near Guj Offset, Vatwa	079-5832846
9.	Shree Prabodhrawal Memorial Trust ,Vanprasthashram Vishwajyot Ashram, Motera road, Sabarmati	079-7571414
10.	R J Trivedi Suvarna Mandal Trust, Vridhashram Nr. Khodiyarmata Temple, satellite road, Post Ambali	--
11.	Jeevan Sandhya, Kasturba Narayandas Kapadia Trust, Nr. Narmada Vasahat, Bhavnagar Road, Dhandhuka Taluka	--

Sr. No.	Names	Contact no.
	AMRELI	
12.	Guru Dattatrey Vridhashram Vridhaniketan, Amreli 364601	--
13.	Dikara nu Ghar Vridhashram Ne. Jivraj Mehta Polytechnic, Lathi Road, Amreli	0279-220735
	ANAND	
14.	Sachhidanand Sewa Samaj Trust Vridhashram P O Box No. 19, Dantali, Petlad, Anand	02692-22480
15.	Shree Ram Krishna Sewa Mandal Anand Vridhashram Opp. Town Hall, Anand	--
16.	Lakhiba Bhagini Pariwar Trust Vridhashram Lahibaa Bhagol, Anand	02692-54646
17.	Shree Ananddham Opp Hanumam Mandir, Lambhel, Anand	02692-54848
18.	Shree Jalaram Sewa Samaj Trust Vadil Vishram Bhavan Opp. Ashok Park, Borsad	02692-23348
	BANASKANTHA	
19.	Vadil Vishranti Gruh Palanpur Banaskantha	53336
	BHARUCH	
20.	Jai Shree Jalaram Bapa Sewa Mandal Trust Vadilo Nu Ghar Nr. Kaasak Kuvara	0264- 245208
21.	Shree Jalaram Bapa Lakashray Trust Ma Bapu nu Mandir Rajendranagar Society, Rajpipala	0264-220974
	GANDHINAGAR	
22.	Kailashdham (vridhashram) Mahudi Road, Post Pethapura, Gandhinagar	02712-78267
23.	Chahana Vridhashram Plot No. 711, Sector 6 B	--
24.	Hariom Vridhashram and Annashetra Post Manekpur (Manasa), Gandhinagar	--

Sr. No.	Names	Contact no.
25.	Swayam Sidhha Old Age Home Lok Kalyan Kendra, Nr. RTO Office, Sector 30	02712-60088
26.	Vadilono Vishamo Vrindavan Dham, Gandhinagar Mahudi Road, Varsoda, Gandhinagar	02712-3241845
	JAMNAGAR	
27.	Manad Mandir, Shri M P Shah Municipal Vridhashram, Aerodram Road, Nr. Khodiya Colony, Jamnagar	0288-673462
28.	Shri Andabava Sewa Sanstha Trust, Shri Sakarben Sunderji Anjariya Mahila Vridhashram Sewa, Limdalane, Jamnagar	0288-676051
29.	Shree Ranjitsinhji Niradhat Ashram Bh. Dr. Bhuvana Na Bangala, Sasekshan Road, Jamnagar	0288-678809
	JUNAGADH	
30.	Manad Mantri Shree Vridhaniketan Narsinh Mehta Chora Road, Junagadh	0285-650597
31.	Manad Mantri Shree Rashtriya Andhajan Sanchalit, Andha Vridhashram Swami Vivekanand School Ground, Junagadh	--
32.	Mohanlal Gordhandas Kotecha Trust Valima Lohana Apna Ghar Porbandar	--
33.	Shreemati Vidyaben Dipchand Gardi Apna Ghar Opp. Sonapura, Bh. Gayatri Shaktipith Bh. Ramwadi, Shantimarg	0285-622085
34.	Brahmanand Suretdham Ashram Via Sarsai, Village Chaparda, Tal-Visavadar	0285-246326
	KHEDA	
35.	Chandlal Madanlal Vanprasthashra Uthkantheshwar	02697-244218
36.	Shantilal Mohanlal Shah Akshardham Nr. Ganesh Talkies, Dakor	--

Sr. No.	*Names*	*Contact no.*
	KUTCHH	
37.	Shree Bhuj Lohana Mahila Ashram Trust Vridhashram, Santosh Society, Nr. V D High School, Kacchch Bhuj	02834-23464
38.	Madhapur Leva Patel Apna Ghar Nava vas Saraswati Vidhyalaya Road, Madhapur Kacchch Bhuj	02834-40317
39.	Shree Thakersi Pragji and Nanabhai Thakarsi Khotari Jivansandhya Old Age Home Sukheri, Post Roha Kotda, Tal-Nakhatrana, Kacchch	02834-89238
40.	Manad Mantri Shree Navchetan Trust, Andhjan Vridhashram, P O Box-30, opp custom Check Post, N H 8A, Bhachau, Kacchch	--
41.	Meghji Sejpal Jain Ashram Nagji Amarsinhji ni Vadi, Mandavi, Bhuj Road	--
	NARMADA	
42.	Manad Mantri Shree, Jilla Bharuch Sewa Sangh Rajpipala, Old Age Home, Mota Piparia Narmada	02640-20023
	NAVSARI	
43	Parsi Infirmary Vridhashram Rustamwadi	–
	PANCHMAHAL	
44.	Nirant Vridhashram, Beside Jalaram Mandir, Vavadi, Godhra Taluka	--
	PATAN	
45.	Smt. Kasturiben Devjibhai Shah Vanprasthashram Arradhana Kendra, Sarwamangalam Ashram, Sagodai Village	02841-22595

Sr. No.	Names	Contact no.
46.	Shree Khemchandbhai A Patel Vridhashram Sander Village	--
47.	Laxmiben Bhudarbhai Patel & Shiviben Narsinhdas Patel Muktidham Selavi Village, Post Palasar, Chansma Taluka	02841-63336
	PORBANDAR	
48.	Vadilono Visamo, Kedarehwar Road, Khiraara Village, Ranavav Taluka	0286-246569
49.	Pujay Valima Lohana Apana Ghar Vridhashram Nr Railway Tracks, Chaya Road	0286-243459
50.	Sewa Ashram Charitable Trust, c/o Shree Hasmukhbhai Nathubhai Buddadev Kedareshwar Road	--
	RAJKOT	
51.	Andh Apang Vridhashram Gandhigram, Raima Road	0281-2240135
52.	Ramik Kunwarba Vridhashram Akhil Mandal Parishad, Gondal Road	0281-2445572
53.	Shree Nilkanth Mahadev Anath Gurukul Ashram Trust, Modi Marad Taluka, Dhoraji	0281-2484038
54.	Jalaram Trust Sanchalit Mahila Vridhashram Malviya nagar	--
	SABARKANTHA	
55.	Smt. Madhuben Vasantlal Shah Shreenathdham Vridhashram, Vasantlal Charitable Trust, Amardeep Co-op. Housing Society Ltd; Opp. Aksharpurshottam Swaminarayan Mandir	--
56.	Sahyog Krushth Yogna Trust Ashakatashram Vridhashram, Rajendranagar Crossing, Himmatnagar	--

Sr. No .	Names	Contact no.
	SURAT	
57 .	Shri Ambika Niketan Trust, Vridhashram Veshu Road, Nr Piplod Health Centre, Taluka Choryasi	0261-222660 09978811188
58 .	Sheth D. V. Shroff Ashaktashram Hospital 7/803, Rampura Road	0261-2422060-61 2422173
	SURENDRANAGAR	
59 .	Manad Mantri Shree Kirchandbhai Kothari Vanprasthashram, Nr Broad Gauge Station, Nr Kasturba Society	--
60 .	Manad Mantri Shree Jivan Jyot Trust Vridhashram, Vagela Village, Vadhwan Taluka	--
61 .	Mantri Vidyapith Manavmandir Building Vanprasthashram, Nivasi Sanstha For Old	--
	VADODARA	
62 .	Manad Mantri Shree Sindhu Sewak Sangh Premdas Jalaram Vridhashram, Swami Premdas Bhuvan, Fatehpura	--
63 .	Jalaram Sewa Samaj Trust, Vanprasthashram Nr Ghelani Petrol Pump, Nizampura	0265-2791793
64 .	Muni Sewa Ashram Vanprastha Mandir Goraj Village, Taluka Waghodiya	02668-268004/5 09974094154
65 .	Late Chimanbhai Patel Vridhashram Village Bamroli, Taluka Sankheda	--

APPENDIX - 6

Nutrition Health Education

A training tool used for imparting education to caregivers as well as elderly for awareness.

Manual for Elderly Health snd Quality of Life

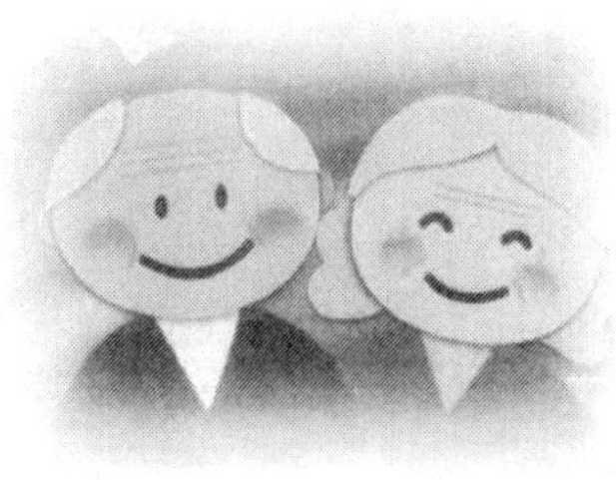

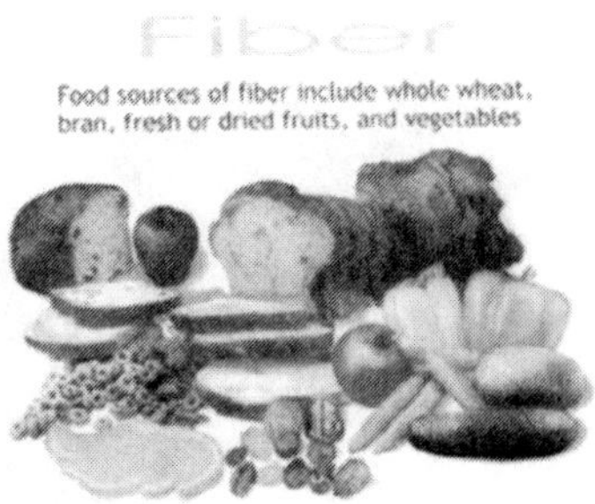
Fiber
Food sources of fiber include whole wheat, bran, fresh or dried fruits, and vegetables

Dietary Tips

- Consume fibre rich foods like whole fruits, green leafy vegetables and whole grains.
- Fiber would help in controlling blood sugar and cholesterol levels and aids digestion.
- Simple carbohydrates be avoided like sugar.

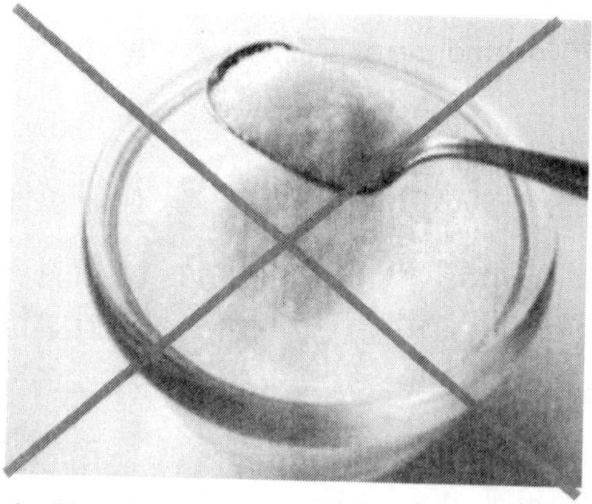

- Vitamin D rich foods like milk and milk products, fish and green leafy vegetables should be included in the diet.

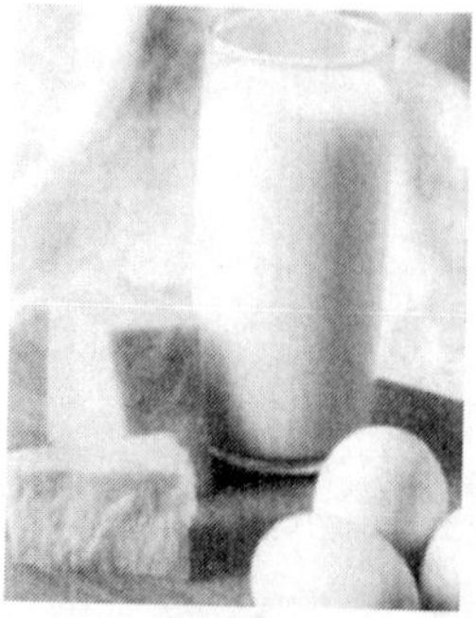

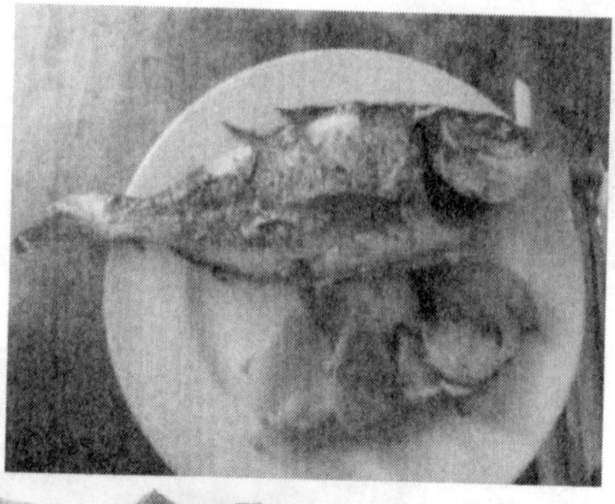

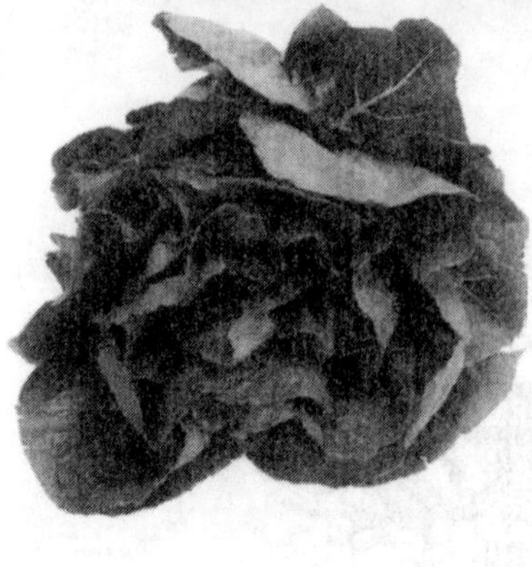

- Use limited amount of salt in cooking.

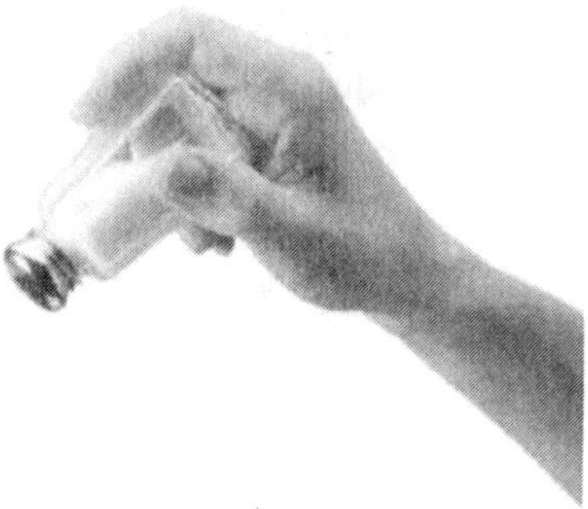

- Include colourful vegetables and fruits in your daily diet.

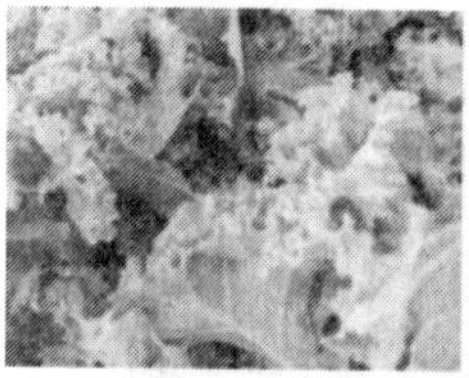

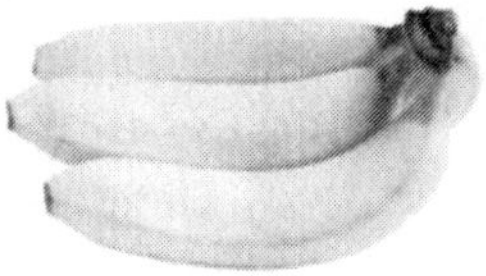

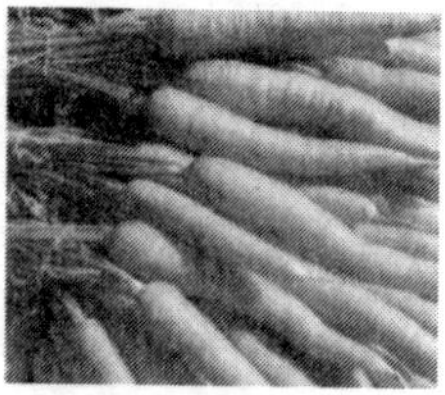

- This has antioxidant properties, which helps to fight against and reduce danger for diseases like cancer.

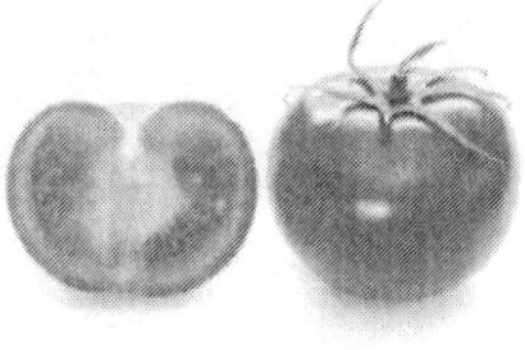

- Proper vitamin and mineral supplement should be given to the elderly regularly as they are more prone to develope deficiencies.

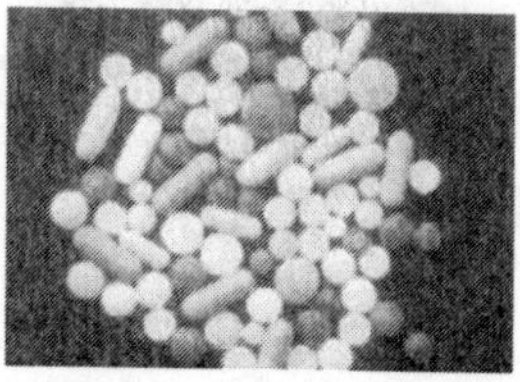

Following signs and symptoms are observed in deficiency of nutrients

(1) Deficiency of Iron (Anemia)

Signs (a) White part of eye turns yellow.

(b) Spoon shaped nails.

(c) Giddiness and tiredness

Food Sources

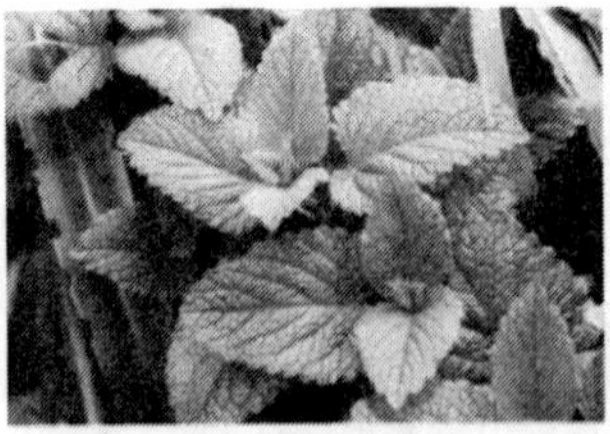

Green leafy vegetables

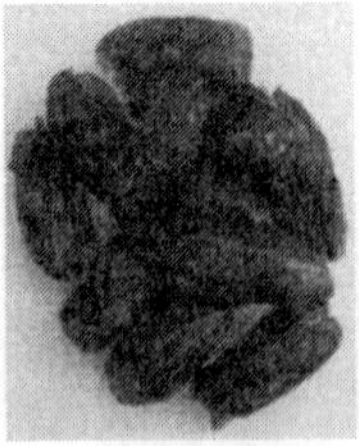

Dates

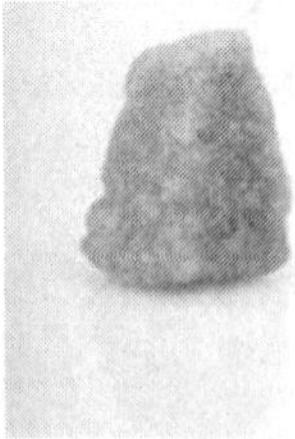

Jaggery

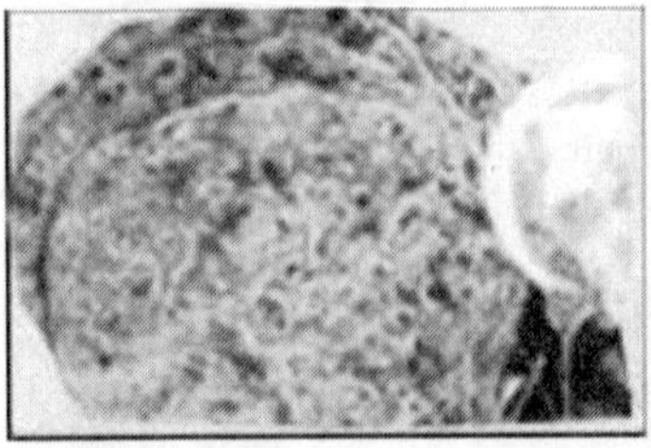

Bajra

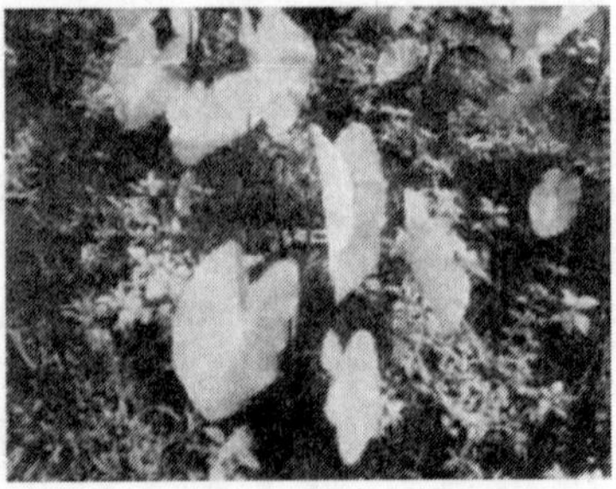

Colocacia leaves

- Consume citrus fruits daily which contain lots of Vitamin C that helps in absorption of iron in the body.

(2) Deficiency of Calcium

Signs:(a) Soft bones.

(b) Bent vertebrae.

(c) Frequency of fracture on falls.

Food Sources

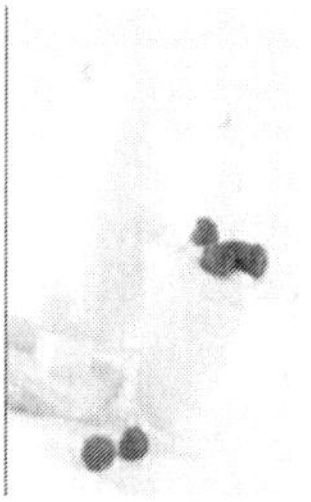

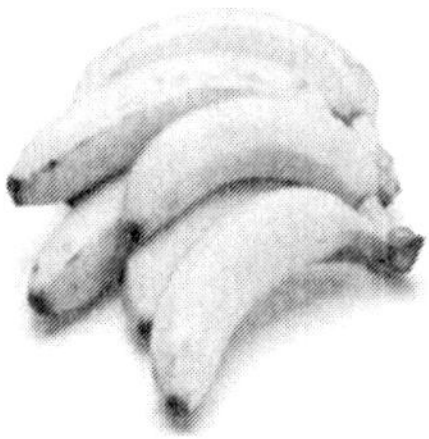

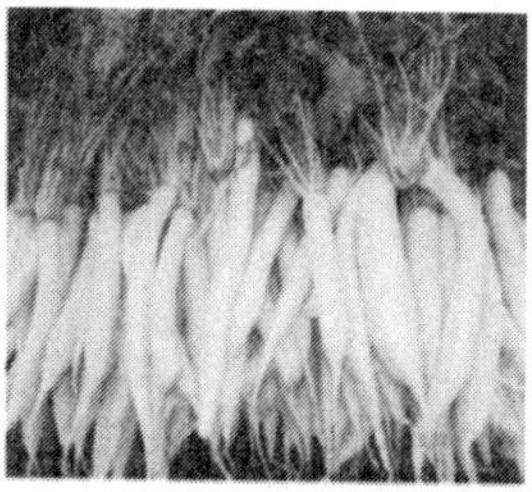

Milk and milk products

Banana, etc.

Raddish greens

- Consume vitamin D daily that helps in absorption of calcium in the body.

(3) Vitamin A DeficiencySigns like

1. Night blindness
2. Vision problem
3. Bitot's spot
4. Corneal xerosis
5. Keratomalacia

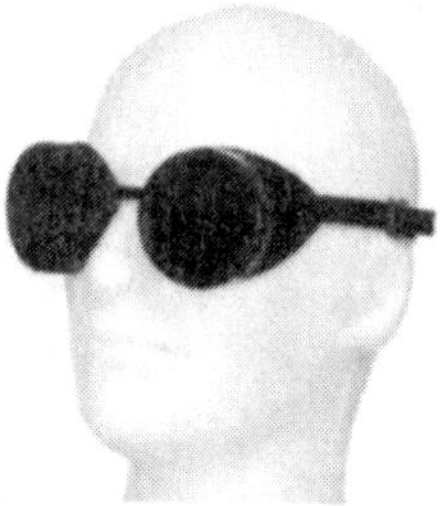

Vitamin A Food Sources

Yellow/orange fruits and vegetables

- Like ripe papaya, mango, Carrot, spinach, etc.

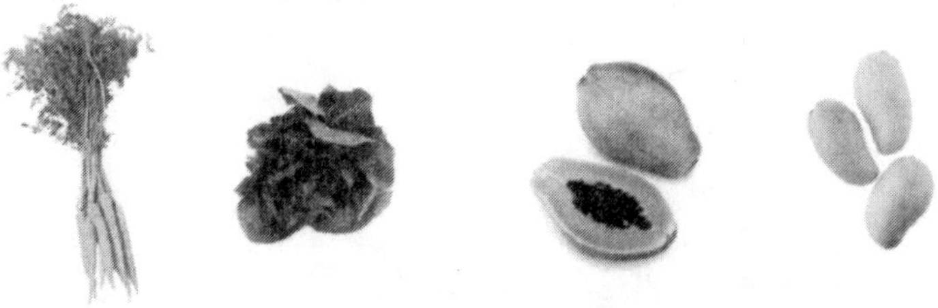

- Oil and Ghee are also good

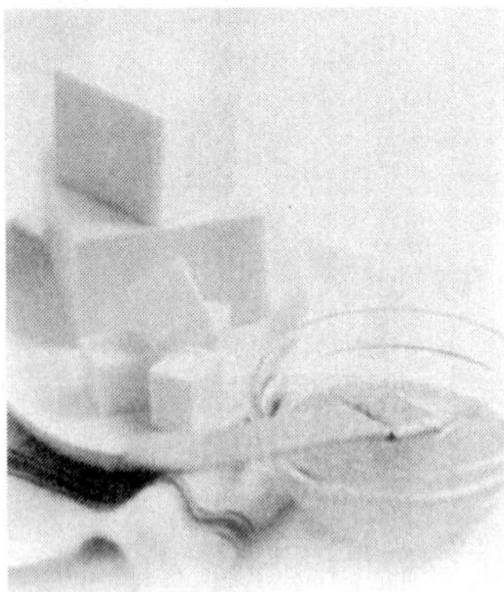

(4) Vitamin C Deficiency Causes

- Infection, esp. on tongue, bleeding gums and lack of healing wounds.

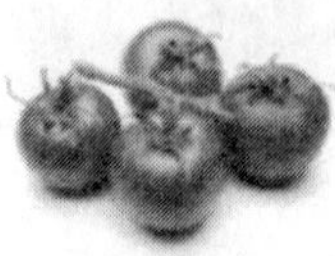
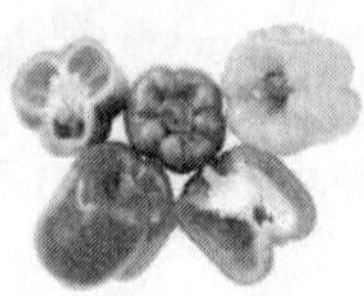
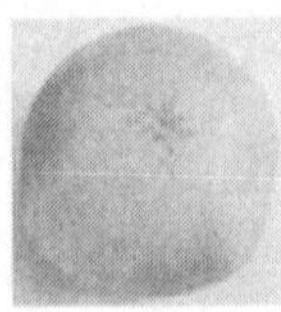
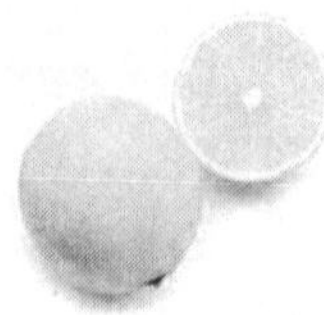

- Citrus fruits like amla, lemon, tomato, capsicum are some of the rich sources

(5) Vitamin B Complex Deficiency Causes

- Dry and itching skin, ulcers in Mouth, cut lips, etc.

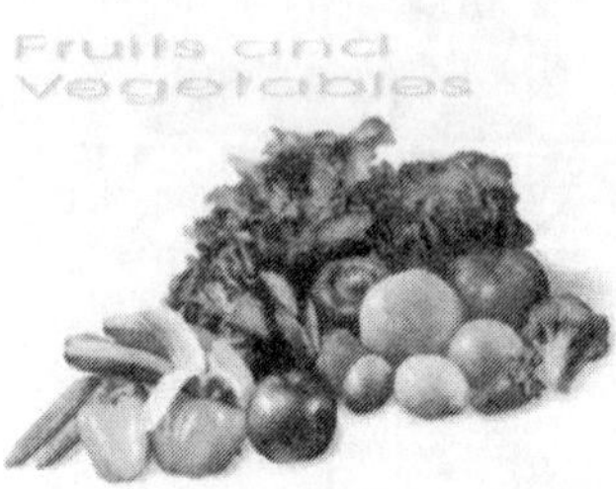

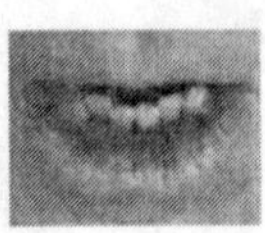
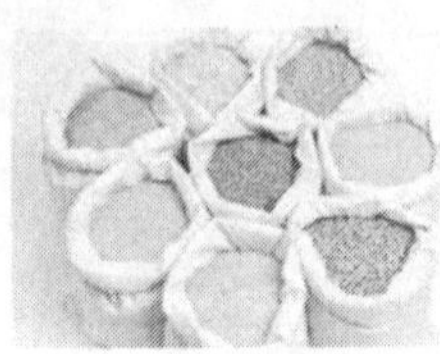

*ADAM

- Whole cereals and pulses, green vegetables and whole fruits contain good B vitamins

Mental Disorders in Elderly

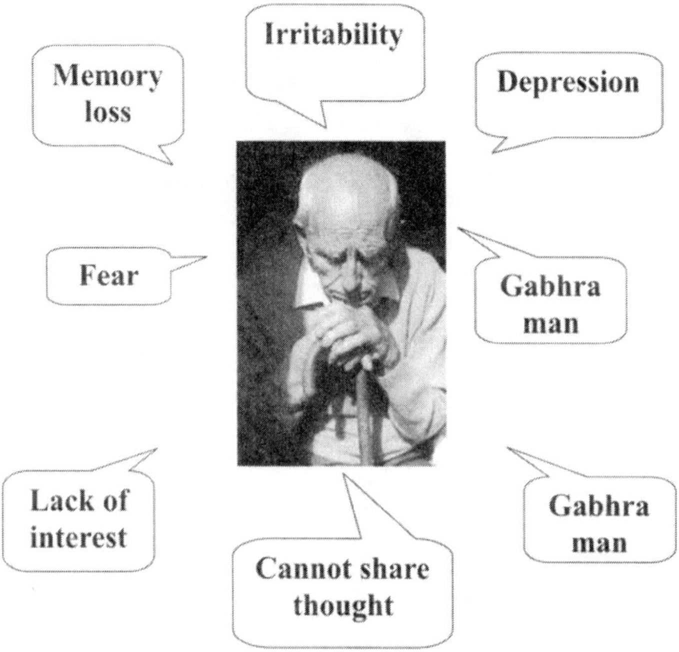

Causes of Poor Mental Health

1. Bereavement of spouse
2. Loneliness
3. Retirement
4. Economic Dependency
5. Poverty
6. Generation gap
7. Physical incapability
8. Adjustment problem
9. Lack of care by family

10. Loss of decision making skill

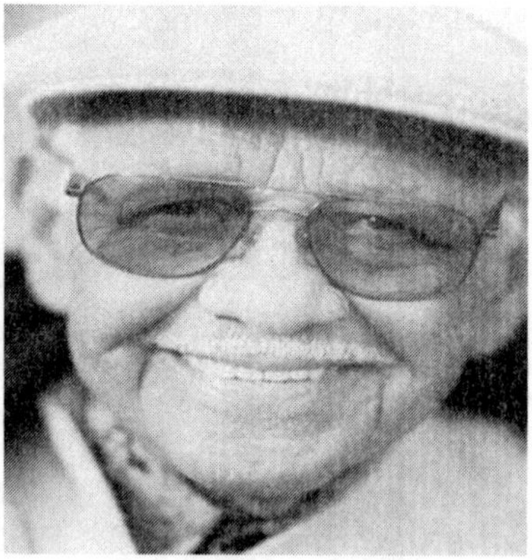

Cure of Mental Disorders

- Care and support elderly
- Take them for outings
- Encourage to do task which they like most
- Have balanced and healthy foods
- Include them in family decisions

Importance of Water in Elderly

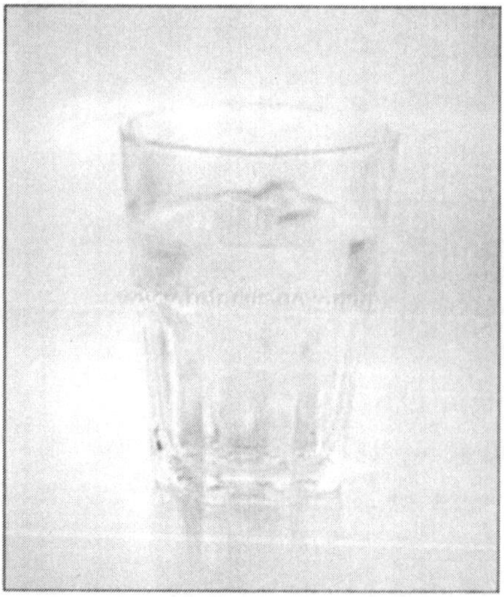

Importance	Deficiency
• Moist skin	• Very tired feeling
• Maintain body temperature	• Feeling thirsty
	• Lack of hunger
• Removal of body toxins	• Breathless
	• Lack of concentration
• Help nutrients transportation	• Feel vomiting
	• Headache, dryness
• Help easy digestion	• Raise body Temp., Yellow urine
• Tension	

Diarrhoea

- During diarrhoea eat food like curd, butter milk and soft foods like - khichdi, rice and dal and food with low oil content.
- Drink plenty of water with sugar and salt.
- Patient should rest properly and maintain hygiene and sanitation.

Parkinson's

- Patient should be given vitamin B complex rich food like green leafy vegetables, fruits and whole cereals.
- Patients should remain involved in daily routine activities, do little exercise and move around.
- Take regular medicines as per doctor's advise.

Dietary Awareness

- Eat little quantity frequently.
- Eat light food in dinner.
- Prefer to drink warm milk before going to bed.
- Eat whole cereals and pulses everyday.
- Eat calcium rich food daily.
- Eat 300- 500 gm of fruits and vegetables.

- Avoid tea/coffee beverages at night.
- Reduce consumption of salt, sugar and fats.
- Take regular meals daily.
- Avoid feasts and fasts.
- Avoid fast foods, processed and canned foods.

Tips for Healthy Living

- Take balanced diet.
- Do yoga meditation and exercise to remain fit.
- Regular medical checkup is must.
- Involve oneself in social activities.
- Reading and religious activity helps in preventing tension and isolation.
- Be positive.
- Maintain cleanliness.
- Avoid addictions.

Sodium Content of Various Foods

high content foods	*moderate content food stuffs*	*low content foods*	*very low content foods*
Bread, Biscuits, Cake, Pastries, Butter, Cheese, Salted snacks, foods containing baking soda, meat, pickles, papad, chutneys, sauces, shell fish, etc..	Cucumber, carrot, raddish, green leafy veg., corn and its flakes, popped rice, rice flakes, red gram tender, tinda, raw tomato, milk, curd, chicken, fish, etc.	Chappati without salt, fruits, ghee, oil, dry fruits, cabbage, cauliflower, honey, ripe tomatoes, peas, onions, potato, etc.	Jowar, rice, maida, tapioca, sweet potato, bitter gourd, lady finger, pumpkin, brinjal, fruits like papaya, guava, orange, etc.

- Follow dietetians guidelines
- Donot use table salt

Beneficial Consumption of Oils for Diabetes/High Blood Pressure/Heart Patients

RDA of fats = 20-25 gms (4-5 tea spoon)

Ratio for mixing of oils (1:1):

Groundnut + Canola

Groundnut + Mustard

Groundnut + Soybean

Groundnut + Sunflower

Groundnut + Safflower

Groundnut + Sesame

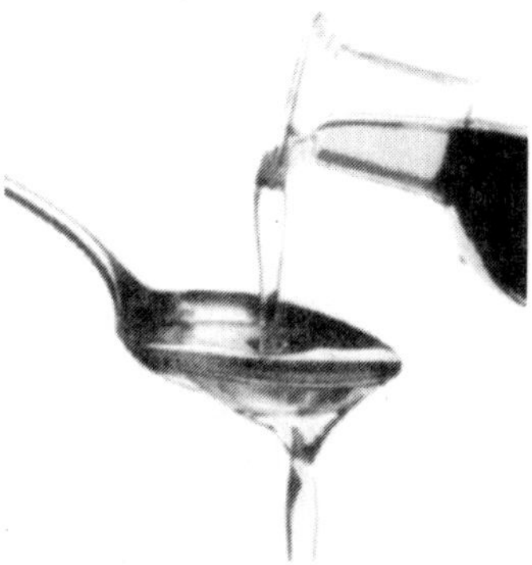

Important Information Regarding Fats which a Person Should Know

- Fat is a Natural Source of Pufa:Mufa:Safa (Pufa) Polyunsaturated Fatty Acid

  Examples: soybean, corn, fish, sunflower, etc.

- (MUFA) MONOUNSATURATED FATTY ACID

  Examples: mustard, groundnut, olive, almond, soybean, sesame, etc.

- (SAFA) SATURATED FATTY ACID

  Examples: ghee, butter, coconut, hydrogenated, etc.

  Dietary ratio in foods: SAFA : MUFA : PUFA = 1:1.5:1

Importance of Exercise for Elderly

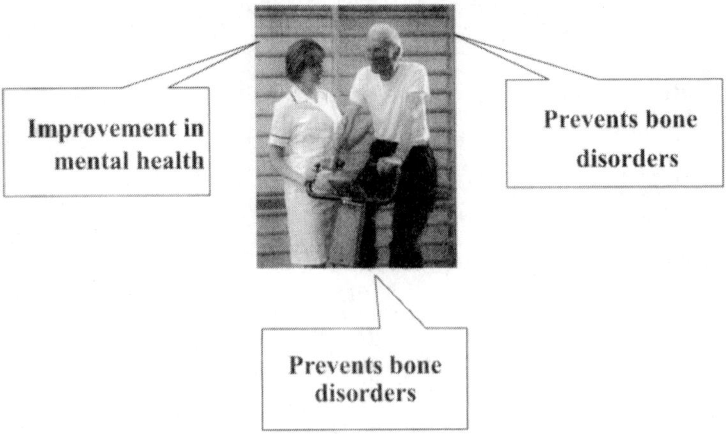

Facts to be Followed Related to Exercise

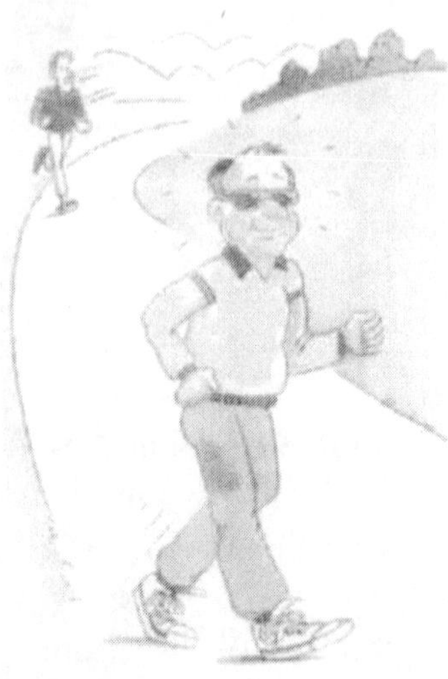

- Exercise 3-5 times in a week.
- For better heart rate exercise 20-40 min.
- Age related diseases like obesity, lung and joints disorder reduces the capacity of exercise.
- Yoga a sanas and walking are the safest exercise for elderly.

APPENDIX - 7

List of Few Anti-agers

Functional Foods

- Foods or dietary components that may provide a health benefit beyond basic nutrition."
- Biologically active components impart health benefits or physiological effects.
- Includes both functional attributes of conventional foods, enriched conventional foods and new food products redesigned with new components.
- Few examples of functional foods which act as anti-agers are:

Sr. No.	*Active component*	*Functions*
1.	**Soybean**	
	Active Components Isoflavones, Daidzein, Genistein, Soluble Fiber	exerts modest estrogenic effects. Improve bone health. Low LDL-C, Low TG, high HDL-C
2.	**Garlic**	
	Active Component-Diallyl sulfide, Allyl methyl trisulfide	Regular consumption reduced risk of colon cancer by 50% Lowers TC by 12-19%

Sr. No.	Active component	Functions
3.	**Fenugreek Seeds**	
	Active Component: Galactomannans, Mucilage gums	Hypoglycemic and Cholesterol reducing effect, contain DHA.
4.	**Flax Seeds**	
	Lignans, Phenols, Flavonoids, Mucilage gums, α linoleic acid & n-3 FA.	Protect the body against inflammations, high blood pressure, lowering cholesterol and triglycerides. Improves the absorption of calcium.
5.	**Garden Cress Seeds**	
	Seeds are rich in iron.	Seeds are used in treatment of dysentery, leprosy, skin and eye diseases, leucorrhoea, scurvy, diarrhea, dyspepsia, asthma, cough, cold etc.
6.	**Wheat Grass**	
	Rich in B vitamins and antioxidants. Best in the form of juice.	Wheatgrass cleanses, purifies and feeds the body by activating the white blood cells, which boost the body's immune system. Wheatgrass juice is also beneficial for people who need to lose weight or cleanse their bodies.

APPENDIX - 8

Common Tools for Elderly Assessment

Nutrition Assessment

There are two possible ways to assess the adequacy of food and nutrition and to detect the presence of inadequacy in food intake among individuals or population groups: the first measures nutritional intake, (Measures of nutritional intake estimate the amount of food a person is eating and can be used to assess adequacy of the quantity of dietary intake) and the second assesses nutritional status, (measuring anthropometric, biochemical or physiological (functional) characteristics that uses objective, measurable criteria that reflect in the changes)

Nutritional Anthropometry

It has been defined as "measurements of the variations of the physical dimensions and the gross composition of the human body at different age levels and degrees of nutrition "(Jelliffe, 1966). Anthropometric measurements are of two types, growth and body composition, and have been widely used for the assessment of the nutritional status of both children and adults. The selection of the ideal single or a combined use of anthropometric indicators depends upon the sensitivity and specificity of the indicator chosen. Sensitive indices are ideally suited for nutritional status assessment in screening or surveillance activities as they are capable of detecting even small changes that occur in nutritional status during conditions of food inadequacy.

Height, weight and BMI are good indicators of nutritional status and the risk of morbidity and mortality in the elderly population. Height can be difficult to measure in the elderly as a result of increasing spinal curvature with age; there are no guidelines regarding the degree of spinal curvature that would invalidate the measurement of height. It can be estimated from knee height or from arm span, although WHO (1995) recommends knee height as being the more satisfactory of the two. The estimated height can then be used to derive BMI, using the recommended cut-off points of <18.5 for under-weight and >25 for overweight,

Weight

- Although weight is extensively used as a nutritional measurement both for assessment and monitoring, its limitations are well-recognised. Accurate measurement requires regularly calibrated and maintained scales capable of accommodating bed-bound people. Clothing, fluid balance including diurnal or monthly cycles, oedema and dehydration, tumor-load and alterations of drug prescriptions are all influential. Weight by itself is difficult to interpret, although change over time may be more informative. Percentage weight change can be calculated. Significant weight loss has been suggested as >5 per cent loss in one month or >10 per cent in six months, although 5-10 per cent loss may indicate nutritional 'risk'. Loss of >5 per cent over one year has been linked with increased mortality (Wallace et al., 1995).

<table>
<tr><th>Classification</th><th colspan="2">BMI(kg/M.Sq)</th></tr>
<tr><td>Screening for obesity/ overweight</td><td>Principal cut-off points</td><td>Abdominal cut-off points</td></tr>
<tr><td>Underweight</td><td><18.50</td><td><18.50</td></tr>
<tr><td>Severe thinness</td><td><16.00</td><td><16.00</td></tr>
<tr><td>Moderate thinness</td><td>16.00 - 16.99</td><td>16.00 - 16.99</td></tr>
<tr><td>Mild thinness</td><td>17.00 - 18.49</td><td>17.00 - 18.49</td></tr>
<tr><td rowspan="2">Normal range</td><td rowspan="2">18.50 - 24.99</td><td>18.50 - 22.99</td></tr>
<tr><td>23.00 - 24.99</td></tr>
<tr><td>Overweight</td><td>≥25.00</td><td>≥25.00</td></tr>
<tr><td rowspan="2">Pre-obese</td><td rowspan="2">25.00 - 29.99</td><td>25.00 - 27.49</td></tr>
<tr><td>27.50 - 29.99</td></tr>
<tr><td>Obese</td><td>≥30.00</td><td>≥30.00</td></tr>
<tr><td rowspan="2">Obese class I</td><td rowspan="2">30.00 - 34.99</td><td>30.00 - 32.49</td></tr>
<tr><td>32.50 - 34.99</td></tr>
<tr><td rowspan="2">Obese class II</td><td rowspan="2">35.00 - 39.99</td><td>35.00 - 37.49</td></tr>
<tr><td>37.50 - 39.99</td></tr>
<tr><td>Obese class III</td><td>≥40.00</td><td>≥40.00</td></tr>
</table>

Cut off points for Waist to Hip Ratio Waist to Hip Ratio

- Measure your waist at its narrowest (usually around the belly-button or just above it).
- Measure your hips at the widest part around your buttocks.

Male	*Female*	*Health Risk*
0.95 or below	0.80 or below	Low Risk
0.96 to 1.0	0.81 to 0.85	Moderate Risk
1.0+	0.85+	High Risk

Diet History

24 Hour Diet Recall

The 24-hour recall method is widely used to provide information on foods consumed by the individual over the previous 24 hours. The quantities consumed are retrieved in the course of an interview that, in the experience of the author, may last from 30 to 45 minutes or more, during which a first free report is obtained without prompts, followed by a prompted report for the purpose of filling in any possible gaps or omissions. The interviewer may use appropriate memory aids, such as photographs of prepared dishes with diverse and calibrated servings, food models, standardised household measures, paper silhouettes of portions or portable scales. Information on cooking methods, recipes, and labels of industrially prepared foods are also retrieved.

Food Frequency Questionnaire

It is the tool to measure food intake most often used in epidemiological research. In its original design, the questionnaire was employed for rating or grading dietary items into four or five categories of consumption for the purpose of differentiating consumers and non-consumers of particular foods and to test for association with disease.

Different variations of the FFQ have been developed, such as those that use qualitative food- frequency scores, or those that provide semi quantitative estimates of the usual diet.

The questionnaire consists of a checklist with a number of individual food items and various levels of food aggregation. The questions relate to the frequency (daily, weekly or seasonally) of consumption of foods or food groups over a given period of time in the recent or remote past. Questionnaires are administered by trained or lay personnel in face-to-face interviews or by telephone, but also may be self-administered through postal surveys.

FFQs have been used alone or in combination with a variety of memory aids such as food models, paper silhouettes, photographs, calibrated household measures and computers.

Sr. no.	*Exchange*	*Approx. amount of raw foods*	*Approx. measure of raw foods*	*Energy (Kcal)*	*Protein (gm)*	*Carbohydrate (gm)*	*Fat (gm)*
1.	Milk	250	1 cup	170	8	12	10
2 (a).	Meat	40	2 pieces or 1 egg	70	7	Neg.	5
2 (b).	Pulse	30	3 tbsp	100	7	17	Neg.
3 (a).	Vegetable A	100	½ cup	Neg.	Neg.	Neg.	Neg.
3 (b).	Vegetable B	100-150	½ cup	40	2	7	Neg.
4.	Fruits	80-100	1 portion	40	Neg.	10	Neg.
5.	Cereals	20	3 tbsp	70	2	15	Neg.
6.	Fat	5	1 tsp	45	-	-	5

Mental Health Status

1. Geriatric Depression Scale (GDI)

Source: Yesavage, 1982-1983.

1. Are you basically satisfied with your life? Yes/No
2. Have you dropped out of many of your interests and activities? Yes/No

3. Do you feel that your life is empty? Yes/No
4. Do you often get bored? Yes/No
5. Are you hopeful about the future? Yes/No
6. Are you bothered by thoughts you can't get out of your head? Yes/No
7. Are you in good spirits most of the time? Yes/No
8. Are you afraid that something bad is going to happen to you? Yes/No
9. Do you feel happy most of the time? Yes/No
10. Do you often feel helpless? Yes/No
11. Do you often get restless and fidgety? Yes/No
12. Do you prefer to stay home rather than going out & doing new things? Yes /No
13. Do you frequently worry about the future? Yes/No
14. Do you feel you have more problems with memory than other people? Yes/No
15. Do you think it is wonderful to be alive now? Yes/No
16. Do you often feel downhearted and blue? Yes/No
17. Do you feel pretty worthless the way you are now? Yes/No
18. Do you worry a lot about the past? Yes/No
19. Do you find life very exciting? Yes/No
20. Is it hard for you to get started on new projects? Yes/No
21. Do you feel full of energy? Yes/No
22. Do you feel that your situation is hopeless? Yes/No
23. Do you think that most people are better off than you are? Yes/No
24. Do you frequently get upset over little things? Yes/No

25. Do you frequently feel like crying? Yes/No
26. Do you have trouble concentrating? Yes/No
27. Do you enjoy getting up in the morning? Yes/No
28. Do you prefer to avoid social gatherings? Yes/No
29. Is it easy for you to make decisions? Yes/No
30. Is your mind as clear as it used to be? Yes/No

Key

Categories	Score
Normal	1-10
Mild	11-15
Moderate	16 – 20
Severe	≥ 21

2. Mini Mental Status Examination (MMSE)

Orientation (Score 1 if correct)

Name this society/building? ---------------
Name the city you are in now? ---------------
What year is this? ---------------
What month is this? ---------------
What is the date today? ---------------
Name the state you are in now? ---------------
Name the country you are in now? ---------------
Which floor of the building are you on? ---------------
What day of the week is it? ---------------

Registration

Name 3 objects and have the patient repeat them. Score number repeated by the patient

Name 3 objects several more times if needed for the patient to repeat correctly. (record trials)

Attention and Calculation

Subtract 7 from 100 in serial fashion to 65 (max. score 5).

Recall

Do you recall the 3 objects named before? ---------------

Language Test

Confrontation naming: watch, pen = 2
Repetition: "No ifs , ands or buts" = 1
Comprehension: pick up the paper in your right hand, fold it in half and set it on the floor = 3
Read and perform the command: "Close your eyes" = 1
Write any sentence (subject, object, verb) = 1

Construction

Copy the design below=1
Total MMSE questionnaire score (Max = 30) ___________

Score	*Categories*
>26	Normal
21-26	Mild
11-20	Moderate
< 10	Severe

Source: Folstein M.F et al. (1975)

3. Cognitive Impairment Test

Item	*Max error*	*Score*	*Weight*
1. What year is it now?	1	------x4=	--------
2. What month is it now?	1	-------x3=	---------
MEMORY PHASE Repeat this after me, Sudhaben Patel 24, Sardarnagar Soc. Nizampura , Baroda.			
3. What time is it? Within 1 hr	1	-------x3=	---------
4. Count backwards 20 to 1	2	-------x2=	-------
5. Say the months in reverse order	2	-------x2=	--------
6. Repeat the memory phase	5	-------x2=	________
		Total=---------	________

KEY:

Categories	*Scores*
Normal	0-10
Abnormal	11-28

Source: Katzman et al., 1983.

References

Folstein MF, Folstein SE and McHugh PR., (1975). "Grading the cognitive state of patients for the clinician". *J Psychiatry Res,* 12(3), 189-98.

Katzman R, Brown T et al., (1983). "Validation of a short orientation - memory-concentration test of cognitive impairment". *Am J Psychiatry* 140(6), 734-739.

Yesavage, J.A, Brink, T.L, Rose, T.L. et al (1982-1983), Development and Validation of a Geriatric Depression Screening Scale: A preliminary report, *Jr Psychia Res,* 17 (1): 37-49.

Index